THE *Thin* FACTORS

A Super Weight Loss Program

By

Prof. Dr. Paul Ling Tai, DPM, FACFS, ABPS, ABAARM

Scientific Research Validated

By

Dr. Steven Morganstern M.D.

Contact info: Doctortai@healthsecretsusa.com

Publisher: United Writers Press, Tucker Georgia 30085

ISBN-978-1-934216-93-4

Limits of Liability and Disclaimer of Warranty

The author and publisher shall not be liable for your misuse of this material. This book is strictly for informational and educational purposes.

Important Warning – Disclaimer

The purpose of this book is to educate and entertain. The author and/or publisher do not guarantee that anyone following these techniques, suggestions, tips, ideas, or strategies will become successful. The author and/or publisher shall have neither liability or responsibility to anyone with respect to any loss or damage caused, or alleged to be caused, directly or indirectly by the information contained in this book. It is advised that you seek therapy under the care of a licensed physician, nutritionist,
or therapist.

ABOUT THE AUTHOR

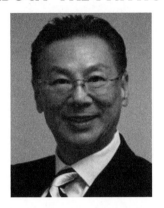

Prof. Dr. Paul Ling Tai
D.P.M., FACFS, ABPS, ABAARM

Prof. Dr. Paul Ling Tai is a trained Podiatric medical physician and double Board certified surgeon specializing in reconstructive plastic surgery of Ankle and foot. He is a member of the Orthopedic/ Podiatric Surgical Reconstructive Team, Surgery Department of the Annapolis-Oakwood Hospital in Detroit, Michigan. He has served under two Michigan State Governors and was recognized with a Vice Chairman's position on the Michigan Board of Podiatric Medical Licensing and as Chief Examiner for new Podiatric physicians. He also served as head of Surgical Residencies. In additional to his various capacities, Prof. Dr. Tai has served as Chairman of the Podiatric Physicians Continuing Education, as well as Chief Compliance Officer for the state of Michigan, supervising doctors. He is also a professor in the New York College of Podiatric Medicine's Department of Integrative Medicine, a professor of AntiAging at University of Paulista (UNIP) in Sao Paulo, Brazil, Prof. Anti Aging at Pontifical Univ. Catholic, Belo Horizonte, MG., a Special Professor of Anti Aging at the University of UNAR, Brazil. Professor of AntAging, Carlos Chagas Institute, RJ. Brasil Co-Coordinator for the Master of Science in Public Health, Anti Aging/Regenerative Medicine. Prof. Dr. Tai is the Official Latin American Delegate for the World Anti Aging Academy of Medicine (WAAAM), and Chairman & President of A4M Brazil. Prof. Dr. Tai is an expert in herbal compound engineering, research and development with Fourteen (14) U.S. Patents credited to his name.

3

A long time supporter, faculty member and lecturer of the American Academy of Anti-Aging Medicine (A4M), American Academy of Asia Anti Aging medicine (A5M), American Naturopathic Medical Association (ANMA), World Organization of Natural Medicine Practitioners (WONMP) and frequent lecturer at countless other Anti Aging & Health Conferences worldwide. Prof. Dr. Tai is also a member of the International Hormone Society and the World Society of Anti-Aging Medicine (WOSAAM). Prof. Dr. Tai is one of the academic contributing authors to the Anti Aging Medical Therapeutic publications published by the A4M and Diplomate - American Academy of Anti Aging Board Certification, oral and written exams. His breakthrough technologies in Natural Health Supplements, Anti Aging Natural Skincare and Proprietary Bio-Hormone Liposome products have been featured in many renowned medical newsletters, television appearances, and radio health talk shows nationwide.

Prof. Dr. Tai is a Knighted physician and the Grand Physician General of the Supreme Council of the Sovereign Medical Order of Knights Hospitaller. He has helped thousands of patients and consulted countless doctors on difficult cases all over the world, earning him the title of the "Doctor's doctor" and "Doctor of last resort". Member of the Royal College of Papal Knights in Americas. Vatican, His Holiness Pope BENEDICT XVI.

Prof. Dr. Paul Ling Tai is the author of the best seller books "Cordyceps Miracles" and "8 Powerful Secrets to AntiAging"; co-authored with Dr. Alex De Souza, MD the new book "Fabulously Beautiful You". Soon will be published this year is his other new book "Noninvasive Plastic Surgery and AntiAging", a textbook co-authored with Dr. Alex De Souza, MD revealing the breakthrough technologies in healthy aging skincare, non-invasive plastic surgery, skin restoration and skin fitness, and latest breakthrough US Patent Weight Loss Technologies.

24141 Ann Arbor Trail, Dearborn Heights, Michigan 48127
doctortai@healthsecretsusa.com

Prof. Dr. Paul Ling Tai
D.P.M., FACFS, ABPS, ABAARM

- Ankle & Foot Surgeon, Orthopedic Surgical Reconstructive Team, Surgery Department Annapolis-Oakwood Hospital, Detroit, Michigan.

- Professor of Anti Aging Master Degree, University of Paulista (UNIP), Sao Paulo, Brazil.

- Professor of Anti Aging Master Degree, Pontifical Univ. Catholic, Belo Horizonte, Minas Gerais, Brazil.

- Professor of AntiAging, Carlos Chagas Institute, Rio de Janeiro, Brasil.

- Special Professor of Anti Aging Master Degree, University of UNAR, Brazil.

- Co-Coordinator Master of Science in Public Health, Anti Aging/Regenerative Medicine. Approved Post Graduates Studies by the Ministry of Education, Sao Paulo, Brazil.

- Official Latin American Delegate and Coordinator for the World Anti Aging Academy of Medicine (WAAAM).

- Founder and Coordinator of A4M Brazil Society and Medical Congress.

- Personal Representative for Latin America to Dr. Robert Goldman, MD, PhD, DO, FAASP- Chairman of A4M.

- Professor of Integrative Medicine. NYCPM, New York, New York.

- Past Adjunct Professor of Surgery. OCPM, Cleveland, Ohio.

- Faculty member, lecturer, workshop, author. American Academy of Anti Aging Medicine (A4M).

MEDICAL BOARD CERTIFICATION

- Fellow – American College of Foot & Ankle Surgeons

- Diplomate – American Board of Podiatric Surgeons

- Diplomate - American Academy of Anti Aging Board (ABAARM): Oral Exam and Written Exam (A4M)

- The Grand Physician General – The Supreme Council of the Sovereign Medical Order of Knights Hospitaller

- Professor, Dean of Endocrinology Dept. University of Natural Medicine, Quito, Ecuador.

- Member - Royal College of Papal Knights in Americas. Granted by Vatican H.H. Pope Benedict XVI, signed by Vatican Secretary of State Cardinal Bertone.

- Chairman & President, A4M Brazil (American Academy of Anti Aging Medicine-Brazil)

OTHER BOOKS BY PROF. DR. PAUL LING TAI

- Cordyceps Miracles 2005

- 8 Powerful Secrets to Anti Aging 2007

- Fabulously Beautiful You! 2009
  Co-Author: Dr. Alex De Souza

- Novos Principios de Cirurgia Plastico Esthetica e Antivethecimento 2009- Co-Author: Dr. Alex De Souza

TABLE OF CONTENTS

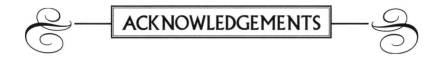

ACKNOWLEDGEMENTS

Special thanks to **Katherine M. Lee** for the important work with this book.

I am extremely grateful to **Dr. Steven Morganstern, M.D.** for his superb clinical work and publications validating the numerous qualities of the Bauhinia.

To **our wonderful patients,** our deep appreciation for your moving stories, courageous commitment, and taking the responsibility for your health. You are the inspiration to our readers!

To the design and the creative work of this book, our sincere appreciation for your talent to **Chezelle Rodriguez**.

- Prof. Dr. Paul Ling Tai

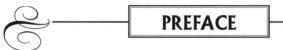

PREFACE

A Message from Dr. Steven Morganstern, M.D.

Life is more than simply living

Life is about using every ounce of power within us. Pain of body or trouble in mind inevitably subtracts from that perspective. My primary focus as a physician has been to restore, as much as possible, that which has been taken away by illness or loss of self-image. These opportunities for empowerment and the resulting joy of having helped advance other people's happiness, have in turn, enriched my own life.

As an urologist I have heard the pain and felt the joy when impotence is resolved and when relationships have been mended. I have celebrated the growing number of prostate cancer survivors and felt a sense of pride in being ahead of the curve in embracing some treatments that are now becoming routine.

I gladly admit that a willingness to look around the corner to see possibilities that lie beyond traditional medical practices has occasionally raised an eyebrow among my colleagues. For example, more than two decades ago, I began to study the physical and psychosexual implications of penile implants in the treatment of male impotence. The restorative benefits in performance and self-esteem…when other medical techniques had proved fruitless…were so evident. As a result, I have since utilized the procedure to return thousands of men to the joy of intimate relations. I was also among the early researchers of Viagra, another important weapon employed against needless suffering caused by ignorance and taboo.

Successful, although with some residual complications affecting the quality of life. I naturally pondered, "What if… I could increase the reliability of palladium seed implants?" I devised and patented the Morganstern Prostate Stabilizing Needle, which steadies the prostate gland during surgery. The device is now widely used and improves the accuracy of the implants, a key to reducing post-surgery complications.

Like most young doctors, during the early years of my career, I concentrated on remedial medicine. Over time, however, I have become increasingly inquisitive about preventative treatments. My brother died from heart disease at age 28. I've always wondered if his passing while so young could have been avoided had we accepted what we now know to be true...that certain diets, herbs and supplements are instrumental in warding off attacks on our health and well-being.

I explored the ramifications of natural male hormone restoration. Success in that area encouraged me to study other natural therapies. The intensity of my studies was recently recognized by induction into the Sovereign Order Knights Hospitaller, an organization devoted to the study of complementary medicine.

Although Bariatric medicine is not my specialty, I desired to play a role in alleviating the calamitous misery of obesity, which is destroying the health and happiness of American men, women and children. Obviously, I am not the first to dwell on the predicament. America is littered with failed diet plans, unused exercise equipment and quick loss elixirs that prove to be the triumph of hope over reality. Several years ago I resolved to remain alert to the possibility that hope for the obese might lie beyond the current boundaries of traditional medicine and misleading marketing.

In the course of research on a possible natural treatment for impotence, I met Dr. Paul Ling Tai, who was concentrating on the same field of study. One day he mentioned exploring the potential of a plant found exclusively in a small, remote plateau in the Ecuadorian rain forest. Possibly, it could have remarkable benefits for the obese.

I had never heard of the plant called bauhinia, and I quickly discovered that there are hundreds of varieties of bauhinia, a beautiful tree with orchid-like flowers. And there are a multitude of natural health remedies attributed to the species. But, only the bauhinia found in a 1000 to 3000 kilometer area of a plateau some 500-800 feet above sea level in the Ecuadorian and Brazilian rain forests had qualities that affected weight loss, apparently with no change in diet or life style and with no side effects.

This book is about our quest to determine the efficacy of bauhinia's properties in the treatment of obesity and about its capacity to balance the connection between mind and body. You will read about the amazing results from blind studies I have already conducted in my Atlanta practice.

In **The Thin Factors,** you will learn about the historical role of bauhinia in Amazonian culture, which is rich in art and prideful self-sufficiency. More than just hope for a better day for the obese, it is a story about possibilities, especially for the economic advancement of natives in this South American country. Natives will be employed to help gather the plants. Others will be utilized in labs built to extract the bauhinia essence that in turn will make it available and affordable throughout the world. Successful employment may even help preserve the rain forest by reducing reliance on logging company dollars.

America is one of the richest, most progressive countries in the world, yet it is not one of the healthiest. Obesity is second only to tobacco as a culprit. Better than thirty percent of Americans are too fat. Obesity-related deaths have climbed to more than 300,000 per year. It is imperative we fight against the current of an increasingly unhealthy society. That is the hope offered by bauhinia.

Steven L. Morganstern, M.D.
February 1, 2009

INTRODUCTION

This we know; all things are connected like the blood that unites us.
We do not weave the web of life; we are merely a strand in it.
Whatever we do to the web, we do to ourselves.
Chief Seattle

I have a passion! I love to teach and share the cutting-edge
information on topics of anti-aging and natural medicine with
my patients and other doctors throughout the world. My fervor
is unusual because I carry the heavy workload of a doctor and
a surgeon. Yet, because I realize I have much to learn, my mind
loves to wonder, explore and create and cannot turn off the flow of
inspiration I receive from my audience, colleagues and patients.

So I've crisscrossed America, Asia, South America and Europe,
and flown to the far reaches of Dubai, Bali and Malaysia. Over
the last several years, every other week, I've traveled by plane to
popular and remote locations. I've covered over two million miles in
commercial flights in just a few short years and sat in small, crowded
airplane seats for twelve to twenty-four hours at a stretch. My every
muscle cramps, my feet swell, I have to monitor my breathing and
keep myself hydrated. People ask me what drives me to do this? An
excellent question indeed!

As I traveled, I've become intensely aware of the changing
human condition by watching the people as they go about their daily
business in airports and in the marketplaces of various countries. I
hear their health concerns.

> *Today's children will be the first generation whose life
> expectancy will be shorter than previous generations.*

I also know there are answers to the health issues that plague the growing numbers of Baby Boomers, their children and grandchildren. Never before have all of us together faced such a challenge for the first time in history.

Please take a moment to think about this alarming possibility for your children and grandchildren. We have grown so used to the progress of medicine that the idea of children living shorter lives than their parents has still not registered. We have so accepted the trend of *Healthy Longevity* that the reality of the situation has not quite dawned upon the majority of people.

Yet, immune system disorders exist to which we have *no definite answers*. There are still recurring diseases of decades past that have baffled us and *do not respond* to modern treatments.

One visible issue that so concerns me in my travels is the growing **Obesity Epidemic. *I am a doctor who sees the global impact of obesity as a disease!*** I hold the issues surrounding it seriously enough to travel and teach and to search for and discover natural solutions!

I talk with other doctors about a variety of topics from mental diseases like Alzheimer's to osteoporosis, severe fatigue and lack of energy, all the way to Metabolic X syndrome and diabetes. We also exchange ideas about obesity, the modern epidemic, from which develop the diabetes, cardiovascular and circulatory symptoms like gangrene of the limb and feet that results in amputation.

I also travel extensively because I feel privileged as a lecturing professor to be invited to speak at universities, medical schools, anti-aging medical society conferences and natural medical organizations around the world. In doing my small part, I always learn more than I teach.

My discovery is, ***"The more I share health and medical information with doctors worldwide, the more I realize what I don't know."*** One natural result is that I learn a great deal from hanging out with some of the brightest doctors on Earth. I am very fortunate!

Precisely in one of those moments of open mind and discussion of natural health information, I met three wonderful doctors, **Dr. F. Pinto, Dr. M. Pinto and Dr. A. Mitrani,** who shared with me amazing information about the different herbs, plants, and botanical extracts from the Amazon. The three doctors were excited about one plant in particular. They called this short, broad bush by the name of ***"healing tree."*** I subsequently learned its proper name as ***"Bauhinia."***

I spent several hours with these three great doctors and then researched on my own to realize that this extraordinary plant demanded further investigation. I soon set out on a personal search for its leaves in the great forest of the Amazon. To do so, I left the modern world with its skyscrapers, crowded cities, and modern air travels to seek answers in the most primitive and primary of venues, the pristine Amazon Forest.

Prof. Dr. Paul Ling Tai, DPM, ABPS, FACFS, ABAARM
February 1, 2009

My Favorite
Success Stories!!!

May all your success stories be GREATER

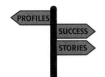

Carlos M.

Weightloss Testimony - February 16, 2010

For the past 10 years several pounds had innocuously found their way onto my body. At first it was no big deal, clothes just fit a little tight. But 3 years ago when I moved to Texas in the winter and my activity level declined somewhat, all of the sudden those few pounds (about 10 at that time) turned into 25 in less than a year! All of a sudden, I had to buy clothes because I couldn't fit into my old suits or pants – I had become fat. Everyone said, Carlos be realistic, after all you turned 50 and that is what is supposed to happen to your body, but I refused to accept it. The problem was that as I tried to work out more as I had in the past, the stubborn fat did not want to come off my body. Also, it was hard to run like I used to at this weight and when I would, my joints and back would ache for days.

It was quite depressing to be overweight but with the larger "new clothes" I covered it up pretty well, except you could really tell on my face. Several months ago my production manager had put a video of a seminar I did in 1995 up on You Tube and when I saw the difference it blew me away and I knew I had to find a way to get back to my ideal weight and body composition.

I spoke to my good friend and doctor, Dr. Paul Tai who I was working with on an anti-aging protocol and with embarrassment told him my "fat" predicament. To my utter shock & amazement which quickly turned to joy, he told me he had lost 50 pounds using this protocol and now had a 29 inch wait (which is exactly what I used to have)!

The crazy thing is that people were always telling

me how I didn't look my age and what good shape I was in. I guess I believed the looking young part as I've always looked young for my age, but the good shape part I didn't buy.

My wife and I had been studying wellness & nutrition for 20 years. I had even trained with a trainer who coached bodybuilding champions in the early 90's. Not to mention, I was an athlete in school.

Over the past years I had used various weight loss/fat loss strategies from Atkins and Protein Power to the Zone to various bodybuilding regimens. While I lost weight and fat with all of them, none of them provided the exact result I wanted and when I gained weight after a while, it was in greater amounts than before and in the wrong places.

When I saw the facts pertaining to Dr. Tai's program, it all made perfect sense, especially in light of everything I had learned about physiology. My wife and I dove into it with 100% commitment and when I lost 10 pounds in the first 10 days, I knew this was the most amazing fat loss program ever. When I started my waist was 35 inches and it is now down to 30 inches. I lost 25 pounds in 30 days and got incredible side benefits... The acid indigestion I'd been suffering from for at least 20 years went away in 10 days. I can now enjoy spicy foods where before I couldn't go near them. Additionally, the mobility in my lower back which I thought stemmed from an injury I had in the early 90's has improved to an amazing degree as I believe that redistribution of fat from bad fat to critical fat has occurred and increased my flexibility and eliminated pain.

I look and feel like I did in my early 30's. There's no question that the science behind this program works!

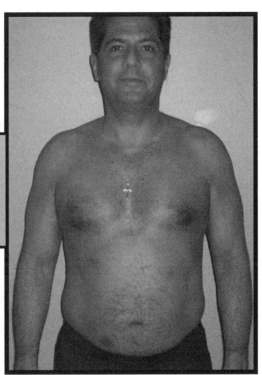

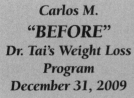

Carlos M.
"BEFORE"
Dr. Tai's Weight Loss
Program
December 31, 2009

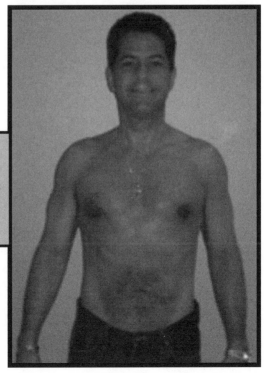

Carlos M.
"AFTER"
Dr. Tai's Weight Loss
Program
February 15, 2010

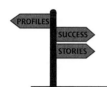

Cecy M.

Weightloss Testimony - February 16, 2010

I'm a 47 year old woman who by everyone else's standard was considered in really good shape. In fact, I was always being asked, "Cecy, how do you stay so skinny?" But the interesting thing was that in clothing I looked fine, but in a bathing suit, I hated how I looked, not to mention looking at myself in the mirror... I was self conscious of my lower body and I was starting to feel like the years were finally getting to me. Not only was I starting to put on body fat in places I never had fat before, but I was not feeling good. I was starting to get arthritis in my right hand whereby I would have lots of pain in my knuckles. I even had a hard time turning a door-knob. I also had pain in my hips and getting frustrated that I wasn't able to workout the same way I used to. This is really what compelled me to do something about my situation. I knew that if I continued doing the same thing, I was going to end up in bad shape.

I was also going through some peri-menopausal symptoms, depressed, no energy, moody, and of course the weight gain so I called Dr. Tai and explained my situation and got on his protocol to regulate my hormones which lead to Carlos' weight gain which lead to his weight-loss program. So my husband and I decided to get on his program and totally commit to doing it 100%!

Let me tell you, I was afraid at the beginning of feeling hungry, getting moody thinking I was going to miss wine and bread... but I never felt hungry. I was actually eating much better than I was before and enjoying it. And trust me, it's not difficult to do. All you have to do is plan your meals ahead and it become a piece of cake, (or not).

*Well, I believe the before and after pictures say it all...
but I started at 125.5 pounds and I am now 112.5. I know for
some people this seams like it's not a big deal, but trust me;
I was the perfect example of a skinny-fat person looking
great in clothes but was definitely carrying fat in places
I couldn't get rid of before. I haven't weighed this much
since I was 17 years old! But the best thing is, you know
when women lose weight, they are fearful of getting saggy...
I know that was one of my concerns because in the past I've
gotten frail looking when I've lost simply 5 pounds. But even
though I've lost almost 15 pounds, my face looks the same
and I do not have saggy skin. And within a couple of weeks
on the program my aches and pains went away! That's
HUGE!!!*

*I love the way I look and feel and I know it's only going to
get better, because I have a new appreciation for vegetables
and how good you feel when you eat correctly. I am really
looking forward to this whole new life style change and
what it's going to do to my health, my looks and my family.*

22

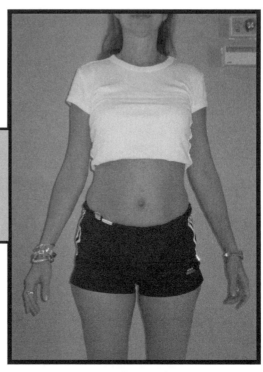

Cecy M.
"BEFORE"
Dr. Tai's Weight Loss
Program
December 31, 2009

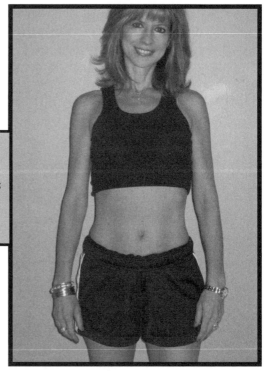

Cecy M.
"AFTER"
Dr. Tai's Weight Loss
Program
February 15, 2010

PART I

WHERE IS THE CURE?

The voyage of discovery is not in seeking
new landscapes but in having new eyes.
Marcel Proust

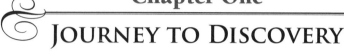

Chapter One
JOURNEY TO DISCOVERY

Determined To Go

The invitation was in my briefcase, and I grasped the tickets tightly in my hand as I walked through a nearly deserted Detroit International Airport terminal. At 10:15 PM, I was exhausted from a full day of unending work, yet excited at the prospects of discovering new cures. I pushed through my fatigue to board the plane and travel to exotic Ecuador.

> *Ecuador is the birthplace of the Amazon River, the mightiest river on the face of the earth. My long trip would take me to an exotic valley of the largest tropical forest, by and large unknown to modern society, called the Amazonian Plateau.*

A full day of work for me usually runs about nine to eleven hours, and while my mind was willing to continue working, my body was not. I settled into my cramped seat, ignored the research papers I intended to read and quickly fell asleep. I dozed, soothed by the white rumbling noise of the plane's engines. Even though the flight was supposed to be an eight-hour trip, the journey seemed interminable. With all of my twisting and turning, I found it nearly impossible to be comfortable within the confines of twenty-four inches of seat.

Inspired By The Vista

I awoke to daylight as it peeked through the window on my right and stared out at the most incredible blue sky with tufted, magically floating cottony clouds. Wiping the sleep from my eyes, I admired a wonderful new terrain below. Before me an unbelievable horizon of green lushness unfolded as far as my eyes could see from an altitude of 30,000 feet.

Coming into my sight was the giant forest, appearing to

take its morning breath, slowly lifting the foggy blanket from its immense green canopy. What an incredible transformation of the botanical world feeding the atmosphere with natural oxygen. This vision reminded me why scientists call the Amazon forest the *lungs of the world*.

The plane landed at Quito International Airport in the heart of Ecuador, and I walked out into a temperate, humid day. I retrieved my luggage along with my briefcase of unread research and went anxiously to meet my ride.

Adventurous Anticipation

My guide was Dr. Montezuma, a naturalist at heart and biochemist by training. He greeted me warmly as natives do in this part of the world. He was the expert who had worked with plants of the Amazon for many years as a botanist-researcher. We shared interests in healthy natural solutions from the Amazon Basin.

Dr. Montezuma whisked me through the city of Quito, full of happy sounds of Latin music, smells of savory spices of fresh cooking. People's Spanish chatter wafted from street cafes and bars. On busier streets the car drivers honked at bicyclists and impatient motorcyclist zoomed loudly around both, spewing a tail of black smoke. Some would call this city of 17th century colonial buildings beautiful with its intricately ornate architecture, situated spectacularly in the midst of the half-dozen snow-capped peaks.

Dr. Montezuma was extremely helpful in describing the practical aspects of the Bauhinia plant and its extraction, but his ultimate job was to take me from the city to the basin of the Amazon. I finally rested well and was eager to leave the next morning after a small breakfast of local strong brewed coffee, freshly baked bread, dried cereals and tasty, local unrecognizable meat.

Onward To The Mighty Forest

We piled our belongings into the battered four-wheel

Jeep and set out on our journey with high optimism. Our destination was a small town named Guayas at the edge of the Amazon forest. From the colorful city, we headed into the country, a hilly landscape full of tall grasses, trees and smaller hairpin curvy, dirt roads.

> *Two hours later, the dirt roads narrowed into an even smaller one-car trail that transformed over several hours into beaten footpaths and rutted gullies. The recognizable road disappeared into a trace.*

Although I am a seasoned, worldwide traveler, I've never seen small trails like these where the rain forest's daily afternoon showers created wide, deep gullies. The driver had to slow to a crawling speed, slower than a walking person. The car so wobbled from left to right, I thought it might tip over. There were times when the entire wheel burrowed into a crevice, and the rocky dirt scraped the metal protective panels of the bottom of our Jeep.

Lush green jungle shaded our narrow road. On the other side was a footpath wide enough for a person on a bicycle or an occasional foot traveler, or people with animals carrying burdens of packages and baskets.

On the rare occasion that we saw another vehicle, we came to a near-stop, slowly passing each other by practically scraping metal to metal, with the trees and branches hitting the car on the other side. On rare occasions, a driver might meet a truck laden with goods piled high, tied down with strings and ropes. The car's driver would wait for the truck to pull over and stop to make room to pass before moving ahead.

Arrival At The Village

When Dr. Montezuma and I finally reached our village destination, Guayail—a tiny conclave of houses surrounding a small white church, we stopped for refreshments and a

bathroom break. Then Dr. Montezuma and I followed a
footpath out of the village leading into the forest. Malnourished
village dogs looking for handouts sniffed at our heels.

We arrived at the native home of Senor Ochoa, who was
introduced to me as a local naturalist, a man who knew his way
around the region and the forest. He knew the village people,
the local mayor and the Indians. Sr. Ochoa was very friendly
with his big smile, but he didn't speak much until it involved
his passion...his medicinal plants.

> He explained that the collections of potted plants in his
> small yard were different medicines for treatment of
> diarrhea, for insulin, for gall bladder and for urinary
> infections. Senor Ochoa had a tremendous, deep
> knowledge of the typical Amazonian local botanies.

Into the Unexpected Rain Forest

After repacking our belongings and loading them into
backpacks, Dr. Montezuma and I followed Sr. Ochoa along a
clear footpath that led into the bends of the Amazonian forest.
We walked deeper and deeper into the forest, and I entered a
vastly different world from how I imagined it would be. The
single footpath required that we walk by carefully placing
one foot in front of the other. The trail wound around natural
objects like huge boulders, or tangled, thorny bushes and
gargantuan trees that could hold five grown men inside where
even the exposed roots where bigger than the trees trunks in
my native state of Michigan. I kept my eyes on my feet because
the tortuous path was deceiving and the surrounding forest was
thick. I certainly didn't want to trip and fall because for sure no
help was apparent anywhere nearby.

First we went around huge bends, then went 180 degrees
to the left, and then jackknifed to the right. So many turns and
bends were disorienting and fatiguing. After hours of following
Sr. Ochoa, this new environment permeated me and left me

exhausted. I shivered with the sheer fear of being lost and left behind. I struggled valiantly to keep up with what appeared to be an easy walk for Sr. Ochoa, but was a difficult tense one for me.

Beautiful Strangeness

Head down, I concentrated on walking around boulders and large, creeping roots. The surrounding darkness startled me when I finally lifted my head and looked around me rather than at Sr. Ochoa's back or at my feet. The forest was dark because of the canopy.

> *The tall trees, like a dark mahogany, stretched up to eighty to 120 feet and formed the uppermost layer that took in the sun and the rain. The thickness of the first layer of canopy ranged from ten to forty feet.*

The second canopy layer was about eighty feet above me. Streams of occasional sunlight broke through it to brighten the misty film that hung over us.

I was also surprised by how noisy the forest was. I have never heard such a cacophony of sounds with birds chirping and squawking, thousands of insects buzzing, monkeys coughing and barking. To the human ear, these polyphonic sounds came together as continuous, dissonant sounds of an orchestra, whose instruments were being tuned in a resonant concert hall before a recital.

The last surprise was how wet and humid it was. We dripped sweat and were sticky from head to toe even though the heat was not overwhelming. **It was a strange, thick atmosphere and was like wearing a heavy, heated wet blanket.**

Chapter Two
The Plant That Heals

> This shamanic view of plants demonstrates the magical "Law of Similarity" referred to by Sir James Frazer in his book The Golden Bough, which states "like attracts like." Thus, the effect of a plant is not just limited to its species; if it looks like another plant of a different species, it will act in a similar way, and if it looks like a human body part or organ, that is what it will heal.

Meeting the Natives

We came to a large clearing after several hours on this foot journey. There were twenty-five similar huts built on stilts, made from woven branches, and covered with leaves and mud. They stood 30 inches off the ground. We stood outside one of them and waited as soft white smoke wafted from the opening in the palm-thatched roof. Small animals like chickens, pigs, and monkeys lived beneath the huts and were tied to the stilts. Children and dogs played freely in the dirt around the area.

A barefoot, middle-aged squat Indian man, dressed in a tee shirt and boxer shorts, introduced himself as Cachiqua (Ka-chee-kwa). He was a Shaman and the medicine leader of this small Indian tribe.

> He was chosen by his father, who was also a Shaman, to be the keeper of the secrets of traditional medicinal plants and sacred rituals with responsibility for the health of the tribal people. Cachiqua served as a counselor, ceremonial head and the tribal medicine man. He was an important man, indeed.

He spoke of the dying art of this knowledge. There was no formal training for passing this knowledge from one generation to another as in his tribe's previous history. He appeared sad when he spoke of not yet having a proper future replacement for himself, as time was not in his favor. Teaching an apprentice takes many years, and he was already getting older with no prospect in sight.

Following the Shaman

For the next several hours I followed Cachiqua around the small streams and crossed with him over rivers. If left by myself, I would never have found the footpaths, which appeared magically in front of him.

He showed me roots that clean teeth and were good for gingivitis. He showed me a type of wood, long branch-like tubes, for detoxifying the liver and the kidneys. He gave me yellow and green fruit called Jabeala to eat, and it tasted sour and slightly bitter, leaving an aftertaste much like spinach does. He showed me magical flowers that would keep the bad spirits away. Much to my amazement, Cachiqua was also very playful.

He showed me a small bush of yellow-green speckled leaves from which a long pod grew. He squeezed it quickly and snapped it, making it explode. He got a kick out of that. His good-humored attitude made this Amazonian Indian man appear to be much younger in spirit than the deep-wrinkled, sunburned face showed in age.

The Healing Tree - Bauhinia

Then Cachiqua came to a medium-sized tree, somewhere around twenty feet tall that had a most interesting leaf.

> *The leaf was shaped like someone glued, back-to-back, two elephant ears in the middle, with sharp pointy earlobes facing each other. The leaf was the size of the two palms of my hands together, side by side. Cachiqua told me that this was called the "healthy tree" because of its dark green color and was wonderful for healing diseases of aging.*

He spoke reverently of the different ways in which he used the parts of the Bauhinia tree for healing. He collected leaves mostly from full-grown trees, and smashed the leaves into a pulp, making a poultice, often spitting to wet it. Then he would place the poultice on the sores and wounds of the legs or arms to draw out infection and to heal wounds.

Another use Cachiqua made of the plant was to place the leaves in an earthen bowl, and mash them with the round end of a stick to break through to the juices. Added to water, this solution was used for bathing babies to clean the sores and infestation off of their backs and tops of their heads. He also boiled the leaves to make a tea for the elders of the tribe to drink, for it was good to calm the blood and improve digestion. *Cachiqua believed Bauhinia is the most powerful anti-aging factor known to his tribe for hundreds of years.*

Another concoction involved leaving the boiling leaves overnight, where the water mostly evaporated. This strong brew extract sat in a bowl for many days to feed to children for eliminating intestinal worms.

I collected as many of the Bauhinia leaves as I could possibly carry in my satchel. Cachiqua said the Indians had been devoted to this plant for hundreds of years, and that he gave his mother a drink of these leaves daily to keep her aging well and healthy throughout her senior years.

> *He spoke of the sacred relationship between these trees and his tribe. He said that Bauhinia has power and mystery, and described how the ancient spirits lived in these trees. During certain nights of widespread diseases among the tribal Indians, one can hear the tree make crying sounds all through the night.*

I was struck by the observation throughout my entire trip to the Amazonian basin that I did not find a single overweight

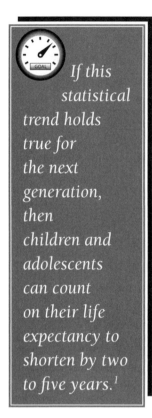

If this statistical trend holds true for the next generation, then children and adolescents can count on their life expectancy to shorten by two to five years.[1]

or obese man, woman or child. Yet, when I gaze out of my laboratory windows in Detroit, two-thirds of all pedestrians walking outside are either overweight or obese.

The obesity epidemic for adults may shorten our current life expectancy by four to nine years. This is an unacceptable tragedy, and I am dedicated to finding a solution.

A Botanical Library

As a scientist with a little knowledge of the Amazonian botanicals, I realized the immense virtual library of chemicals that could come from these millions and millions of forested acres. All you have to do is look back at the key ingredients that the pharmaceutical companies adopted in the last hundred years, from quinine to muscle relaxants and steroids, antihistamines, antibiotics and lately even cancer drugs. Current studies are being conducted for diabetes, anti-inflammatory, antiAging, arthritis, and anti-parasite medications that come from Amazonian plants. These only hint at the infinite myriad of possibilities.

More than a hundred pharmaceutical companies now spend billions of dollars doing research. Governments all over the world hoard the massive species of plants they investigate as they fund projects to unlock the mystery and the hidden power of these compounds. What a travesty that multi-syllabic degree scientists in ivory tower universities believe that men, like Cachiqua, dabble only in *"hocus-pocus"* and *"witchcraft."* I am saddened by this arrogant attitude.

---

[1] Olshansky, S. J. et al. "A Potential Decline in Life Expectancy in the United States in the 21st Century." New England Journal of Medicine, (3-17-2005) Vol 352:1138-1145.

Shaman and Healer

Humbled and awed, I was standing shoulder-to-shoulder with a Shaman and a healer, learning from his wealth of history and healing. Many modern doctors and scientists would consider him uneducated, with little real knowledge of botany and plants, let alone medicine, opting for double blind clinical research of 50 to 100 subjects. The doctors are ignoring generations of daily, positive result-focused human experiences that help resolve illnesses that have existed from the time of our great-great grandparents to kids today. This we call modern science!

Meanwhile, I was thrilled. I was as excited in my 62-year old body as if I were a young kid playing with a brand new toy. Bauhinia was like my toy, and Shaman Cachiqua my new playmate in our multimillion acres of green playground was our sandbox.

I had traveled far to enter a radically different world to seek the help of an Indian curandero whose gifts had been handed down through hundreds of years. Cachiqua's great, great, great, great grandfather was preparing healing herbs in the same way when America was discovered. What respect I have for him, his culture, and his wealth of medical knowledge. I am truly humbled.

Our Botanical Wealth Is Disappearing

The rainforest in our small world has shrunk so much in the recent years. It used to cover fifteen percent of the Earth's surface, and now, *merely five percent is left.* Deforestation, timber cutting, and burning of these marvelous natural treasures cause our botanical wealth to disappear.

> *In less than 50 years, we have lost over 50 percent of our world's tropical forests. Just imagine, every single day we lose another 200,000 acres of rainforest because someone burned it down. That is over 150 acres every minute of every day.*

Some scientists are desperately trying to save the forest because, at this rate, we will have no more forest in another 40 years. I heard the worst news recently: *According to a report from Brazil's National Institute for Space Research, Amazon deforestation jumped 228 per cent in August 2008, when compared to the same month last year.*[2]

The loss continues, as we are aware that **over 150 species of plants, insects, and animals disappear from the face of the Earth every single day and become extinct by** the loss of these great vast forests as their habitat. It is believed that in this part of the Amazonian basin, where the birth of the great Amazon River gathered strength, over 1,500 species of plants are used for medicinal purposes and curing human conditions.

I ask you, "Where will future mankind turn if he has destroyed this spectacular natural resource?"

---

[2] (http://exitstageright.wordpress.com/2008/10/02)

Part II

WHAT INFLUENCES BEING OVERWEIGHT OR OBESE?

Chapter Three

SUPERSIZE SURPRISE

Supersize It!

"I'd like a cheeseburger please."
"Would you like that supersized?
"Can I supersize that for you?"

If we asked for a McDonald's burger or fries in the mid-1990s, the friendly face behind the counter asked us the supersize question. Of, course, we said yes. Who wouldn't want more for the asking?

They could eat more and then not appear gluttonous as they munched in the dark and enjoyed their favorite movie. Silently, they poured it down and put on the pounds.

When the theaters' marketing manager, Wallerstein, became a McDonald's executive, the supersize concept moved through the McDonald's franchises and became an overnight smash. Supersize flourished as other fast food chain enterprises soon presented their unique version.

The concept of *"more was better,"* coupled with psychological pleasure, rewarded our sense of entitlement. The result of more than a decade of this marketing has been an unhealthy combination of overeating and overwhelmed digestion.

The supersize concept was the brainstorm of David Wallerstein, who discovered that people who purchased popcorn and drinks before entering the movie theater seldom returned for seconds. They would, however, gladly pay for a larger size if they paid only once.

Excessive Excess

> *Supersize exploded into excess as we've learned unwittingly to eat more. This has produced an unfortunate result since stomachs expand to accommodate whatever volume is stuffed into them.*

The result, as pointed out by writer Liz Monte, is expanded waistlines. In her article, "Portion Size, Then and Now,"[3] she clearly points out the consequences of the cultural phenomena of supersize, and it is not just that our waists are growing. The servings keep growing as well.

FOODS	TWENTY YEARS AGO	TODAY
Pizza	2 slices **500 calories**	2 slices **850 calories**
Cup of Coffee	Coffee + milk + sugar **45 calories**	Grande café mocha, 2% milk and whipped cream **330 calories**
Popcorn at the movies	5 cups **270 calories**	Tub = 20 cups **630 calories**
Bagel	3-inch diameter **140 calories**	5-6 inch diameter **330 calories**

The once large 20-ounce soda is now 42-ounces; 7-Eleven's 32-ounce Big Gulp has grown into the 64-ounce Double Gulp. In 1996, Starbucks dropped their 8-ounce small cup of coffee and replaced it with the 20-ounce Venti. Even restaurants have substituted the once-standard 10.5-inch plate with the 12.5-inch plate. More is better, right?

Excessive Leaves Us Empty

Imagine if all of this wonderful supersized food was nutritious and contained enzymes, vitamins, antioxidants, and micro-minerals to fuel our metabolism. Imagine how energetic and alive we could feel if the food was real! We can tell

---

[3](http://www.divinecaroline.com/article/22178/49492-portion-size--now)

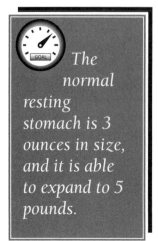

The normal resting stomach is 3 ounces in size, and it is able to expand to 5 pounds.

something is wrong when we are eating and feeling worse rather than better.

Since the excessive calories are empty, we might as well have eaten the cardboard container rather than the popcorn inside the tub for all the nutrition we received. One large tub of popcorn contains the mind-boggling sum of 100 grams of fat, or the equivalent of more than six cheeseburgers.

That tub full of buttered carbohydrates is about 1300 calories, almost a full day's intake for a dieter.

Many of us think that we will buy the tub of popcorn, share it, and not eat all of it. If you can do this, bravo to you! You are the exception. The majority of us don't stop eating. A study from the University of Illinois at Urbana-Champaign showed that people who were given big buckets of popcorn ate roughly fifty percent more than those given smaller buckets.

Professor Brian Wansink's research showed that people will still eat more and are not aware that packaging and fancy branding influence their eating habits. (www.foodpsychology.com)

Wouldn't it be nice if those calories empty of nutrition were actually empty calories? As you now know, they aren't. Their true nature is that while they have no nutritional value whatsoever, they are addictive and loaded with calories. Then too, the biochemical effects on moods are detrimental to your health in addition to the extra calories.

- *One 20-ounce bottle of soda is the equivalent of pouring 17 teaspoons of straight sugar into our bodies!*

- Women who drink one soda a day increase their chances of developing type-2 diabetes by 85 percent. It is like inviting premature aging into your life.

- The soda content of high fructose corn syrup can increase mood swings and energy highs and lows. Mood management and focused activity become difficult at best.

- Combine the high fructose corn syrup with the acid in the drink, and you have a recipe for degrading tooth enamel and tooth decay.

- Another study published in *The Journal of Clinical Endocrinology & Metabolism* in 2004 looked at the metabolic effect of high fructose corn syrup. The results were that after consuming meals rich in high fructose corn syrup, **subjects showed decreased levels of leptin… one of our key appetite regulating hormones.**

DOCTOR TAI'S IMPORTANT TIP

Healthier drinks than soda, especially diet soda, are available. They quench thirst, do not contain the sugar load and are better for your waistline. Healthier drinks include five to eight glasses of water or tea each day for hydration. If you work out or are sensitive to heat or sweating, include drinks with electrolytes to restore nutrients. However, my personal favorite is the world's most perfect drink…natural green coconut juice and brewed iced tea. Some people prefer green tea…your choice of course.

The most perfect electrolyte drink is raw green coconut water because it contains all the necessary ionic minerals and micro-minerals, with the right amount of physiological vitamins and amino acids. This drink is so perfect, in fact, that doctors say in jest that you can open the green coconut top and inject it directly into the veins…of course that would be crazy, but the humor illustrates how perfectly nourishing and compatible the drink is to the human body.

Satisfying the Lizard

Writer Patrick J. Kiger humored readers in his article, "Living Ever Larger: How Wretched Excess Became a Way of Life in Southern California" (*Los Angeles Times*, June 9, 2002). Kiger explained that the desire for excess comes from our most primitive brain structure, the reptilian brain.

> *"The reptilian wants to grab as much food as possible, to be as big and powerful as possible, because it's focused on survival. When it comes to a choice between the intellect and the reptilian, the reptilian always wins."*

Most likely, we will never be able to satisfy the inner lizard, and I wish it were as simple as the evolutionary human grabbing the largest portion. How can the average person say no to supersize campaigns funded by the millions to entice a consumer to *eat...buy...be entitled...gain more...eat?* You see how this requires the strength of your will to say no and stick to it!

On the evolutionary scale, our bodies were designed to handle starvation. Our bodies don't do well in handling excess calories.

The body isn't like a glass that when filled to overflowing simply spills the overload. Instead, bodies store what they can't get rid of. *The result is obesity and its health complications.*

When the Supersize Gets Personal

Most therapists will tell you not to take life so personally, and advertisers will say, "Hey, we're just doing our jobs. You don't have to eat that or buy this." For the sake of your health and your children's health, it is time to take a stand. *Take obesity personally! It will kill you if you don't!*

In the next chapter, you'll learn how serious and widespread the problems of the supersize generation are becoming. The statistics and stories are frightening because they foretell of diminishing health with shorter, more uncomfortable
life expectancy.

Surgeon General Dr. David Satcher calls obesity an American epidemic—a sudden widespread disease. I believe it to be pandemic, becoming more so and fueled by growing, prosperous waistlines. In the next several chapters, pay particular attention to how the waistline has become an important predictor of your health and longevity.

Chapter Four
THE AMERICAN EPIDEMIC

To say that merely by consuming too many calories causes obesity is like saying that the only cause of the American Revolution was the Boston Tea Party.
Adelle Davis

Price of Prosperity is Peril

Peter C. Whybrow, author of American Mania: *When More Is Not Enough*, says, "the more mobile we are, the less active we become." He confirms that the **American mind-set is stuck on more is better. Bigger is better. More and bigger equal prosperity.** This mind-set is wreaking havoc with our health and well-being.

The health issues are being overweight and being obese, but what is the difference in the terms? The definitions for overweight and obese still rely on the Body Mass Index or BMI, which correlates one's height and weight measurements. *To calculate your BMI...*

- *Determine your height in inches and multiply it by itself (ex. 66 x 66 = 4356).*

- *Divide your weight in pounds by your height calculation (ex. 145 / 4356 = 0.03328).*

- *Then multiply this result by 703 (ex. 0.03328x 703 = 23).*

- *This should give you your BMI (23) and you can review the rating scales as provided by table, which classifies BMI levels.*[4]

---

[4] http://www.obesityfocused.com/articles/about-obesity/definition-of-obesity.php

WEIGHT CLASSIFICATIONS	LEVELS OF BMI
Underweight	Less than 18.5 kg/m2
Normal	18.5 - 24.9
Overweight	25 - 29.9
Obesity (Class 1)	30 - 34.9
Obesity (Class 2)	35 - 39.9
Morbid Obesity	Above 40

The National Health Institute's statistics show that two of three Americans are overweight or obese. Data is based on surveys conducted between 2001 and 2004.

- 68.3 million overweight: 29.8 M women and 38.5 M men

- 61.3 million are obese: 34.7 M women and 26.6 M men

- Total is 129.6 million Americans[5]

The Center for Disease Control has equally alarming statistics, which shows that children have increased their weight at the rate of 300% since 1980. **Currently, 77% of our children are overweight and 17% are obese.**

[5] http://win.niddk.nih.gov/statistics/index.htm

DOCTOR TAI'S IMPORTANT TIP

Few people know that the amount of food you eat is more important to weight control than what you eat and how many calories you count. Here are some good reminders that keep the pounds off because eating specific portions satisfy hunger, do not stretch the stomach abnormally, and make digestion more efficient.

When dining out, eat one half of the meal, which normally satisfies hunger, and take the other half of the meal home. This holds true for salads, sandwiches, steak, soup or pasta. If you do not take it home, then give yourself permission to leave the food on the plate.

A socially gentle way I personally use is to separate half of the food to a clean plate. Then I offer to all my friends at the table a morsel taste of the exquisite dish, and I get their comments. It's fun, extremely friendly, and it saves you from eating it all.

Hold these visuals in your mind as you see and feel how much one food serving for weight conscious persons is like:

Carbohydrate like cooked pasta, rice, potato = one-half cup

Vegetables or leafy salad = 1 cup or the size of a tennis ball.

Cooked meat or fish = one-half a CD rom

Snack foods = one handful, then put the rest away

Yes, the statistics are alarming. Yet, are they enough to move us to action? **Most likely not because the more pounds we carry, the less we want to move and act.** We are stuck in that conundrum, and up until now, we didn't really know *help is finally here!*

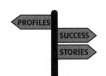
Joe's Profile

Joe grew up in a small Nebraska town where everyone knew everyone, whether friend, family or extended cousin. Joe married his high school sweetheart and settled into comfortable small-town America to raise three children.

Joe was a strong man on the high school football field and physical muscle and dexterity had earned him sports honors. Upon graduation, his brute strength would earn him a living. Over the years, Joe worked construction or did some trucking. Whatever the job, he rose at 5 AM and met his local cronies at the diner for his daily breakfast of hot cakes, eggs and bacon or sausage. Lunch was also convenience food on the road, and he had a balanced dinner with his family at night. Joe gained weight through the years, but kept obesity on the edge with the physical requirements of his jobs. After an early retirement due to back problems, he became obese, especially in his abdomen and weighed 220 lbs. at 5'8".

During his physical checkup at age 60, the doctor found his arteries to be clogged, and intervened with a quadruple bypass surgery. Intestinal surgery followed six months later.

Joe is not an isolated case. Joe actually represents the situation of many working men in America who do not seek medical help, especially for obesity, despite their doctor's warnings that being overweight is a health risk. Each of us has our own blind spots, and the next several chapters will open your eyes to the new scientific evidence-based solutions!

> We know that Americans spend $33 billion dollars annually on weight loss products and services. We don't know exactly what weight loss programs, practices or exercises people employ. A National Health Institutes' survey of 32, 440 persons,[6] representing the United States adult population showed the following strategies to be more popular:
>
> **Eating fewer calories**
>
> **Eating less fat**
>
> **Exercising more**

Only one-third of those interviewed were engaged in or trying those top three strategies. Despite the seeming lack of participation, people are actually desperate for an effective remedy to the problem of obesity, and here's why.

A study showed that the body might suffer a blockage of communication between the brain and the signals sent by the neurons of excess fat storage. Since the brain does not realize the problem of excess fat storage, the brain makes no effort to signal the body to decrease appetite. [7] *So the person keeps the habit of eating and eating. No wonder majority of the people failed with their diet plan!*

Facts on Fads

Diet books are nearly always on the top of the best seller lists right along with cookbooks. A lot of us have tried one or several of the following diets, some of which were more fads than effective, and others with a solid base of evidence.

[6] Kruger J. PH.D. et al. "Attempting to lose weight." Am. J. Prev. Med 26.5:402-6

[7] Swaminathan, Nikhil. Blind to Blubber: Brain May Be Unaware of Body's Excess Fat Stores. Scientific American, 03-08-07).

Grapefruit diets: The grapefruit diet or the Hollywood diet is based on the premise that a grapefruit enzyme aids in digestion of protein. For this diet, grapefruit sections or grapefruit juice accompanies calorie foods of meat and vegetables and 64 ounces of water daily. The drawbacks are that people get tired of eating the same food and experience taste fatigue.

Cabbage soup diet: Cabbage soup is a high fiber liquid with healthy ingredients which clean out the colon. The dieter eats soup with a variety of fruits and vegetables over the seven days of the prescribed diet, which addresses different tastes. Following this seven-day diet would result in loss of weight, most likely in water loss and bowel cleansing. People use this diet to prepare for more serious dietary regimens. Those on this dietary regimen quickly tire of tasteless cabbage, regain the weight lost, and then want to eat!

Raw food diet: This popular diet allows for juicing or blending of fruits and vegetables, but no other preparation of raw food. This vegan diet allows the natural enzyme in the food to help you digest, assimilate and detoxify. Enzymes fuel the metabolic processes in our body, so one would feel more vitality. One drawback of this approach is the high glycemic index of fruits and vegetables. A second drawback is the total lack of protein for a large protein eater.

Atkins diet: This highly popular fad is based on the premise that the body burns carbohydrates and fat as energy. Cutting down on carbs then, one supposes that the body will burn the body fat when carbs are not available. The intended result is a significant drop of pounds.

South Beach diet: Developed by Dr. Arthur Agatson, this diet provides people with knowledge about choosing the right fats and the right carbs. The benefits are lowered cholesterol, more energy and promises a lower risk of heart problems.

New Help Please!

Science Daily (July 2, 2008), reported that the American Heart Association suggested a Population-Based Prevention of Obesity programs. The idea would be that local people lose weight together if they had different levels of adaptations or interventions in the local environment. This is based on the premise that environmental social structures and geography contribute to health habits. These changes could include local intervention clinics, the location of fast food chains, changing types or portions of food served, and building adequate exercise areas… Knowing that our community has local walking trails, dog parks, or biking routes, we could energize ourselves with friends or pets.

What research explained is that our bodies don't have a sense for managing excess, especially food. If the brain becomes blind and insensitive to our excess body fat stores, then we need tremendous discipline to lose weight.

Or we need a therapeutic agent like The Thin Factors Bauhinia to awaken and cleanse the receptors of the brain and affect some biochemical changes to prevent fat build-up. Here is a report on Margie's progress

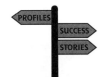

Margie's Profile

*Margie: At age 48, Margie was being treated for hair loss and the new hair was growing in gray. After taking bauhinia, which the indigenous groups of the Amazon use as an anti-aging tonic, she noticed the hair was darkening into the lustrous brown color of her youth. She also lost twenty pounds in eight weeks, going from 137 to 117 pounds and dropping two inches from her waistline and hips. She reported, "Bauhinia has curbed my appetite and given me lots of energy. My husband jokes that he has back his "PYT"—pretty young thing. I went to a family gathering, and my family was amazed at how much weight I have lost within such a short period of time. Now my sisters are asking me about **The Thin Factors**. This is awesome!*

Meantime, overweight and obese people are struggling with their defective receptors and biochemistry in addition to unrealistic expectations from Hollywood influences and tabloid rhetoric of quick fixes like "Lose 15 lbs in 15 days" and "Never diet again."

The Hollywood influence is pretty dazzling in its deleterious effect. Celebrity weight gain is a spectator's feast as we guess who has gained weight while pregnant, lost weight, had cosmetic surgery and which antidepressant medications have side effects of weight loss or gains. The yo-yo effects that we watch a super star like Oprah go through don't show the pain on the psyche, heart, the intestines and body.

A *Yo-Yo* diet is the weight change that occurs when you reach your desired weight loss, **only to put it back on a few months later!** Plus a few additional pounds for punishment.

DOCTOR TAI'S IMPORTANT TIP

Regarding your food in a diet plan, concentrate more on cutting out the carbs and sugar, changing from Colas and orange juice to iced tea, switching from cakes and cookies to strawberry yogurt and sugar-free apricot jam, from potatoes and spaghetti to garlic mashed cauliflower and 5-minute spaghetti squash with tomato sauce.

Refrain or Regain

The *New York Times* published an article, "Commercial Diets Lack Proof of Their Long-Term Success" (November 24, 1992) by Elizabeth Rosenthal. The article explained that diet programs, which have sold weight loss answers for years were pressured by Federal Regulators to start researched-based data about the success of their programs. The meager available data showed that people, who do follow a commercial diet and lose weight, will surely regain their losses as the statistics indicated.

A. One-third of their lost weight regained after one year,
B. Two-thirds or more regained after three years and
C. Most, if not all, in three to five years.

This is discouraging for those dieters, who have put forth the money, time and energy. The writer, however, made a great point. In the same article, Dr. Robert Hoerr, director of medical affairs for nutrition branch of Sandoz Pharmaceuticals, Minneapolis, said sadly that *the weight loss industry is a culture about drugs and food sales, not "a culture of care."*

You have to establish a ***culture of care for yourself.*** Look out for number one—***YOU***—since no one else will do it for you. A culture of care works and the weight will stay off, with the help of specialty supplement solutions discussed in this book that *assist our body's biochemistry to restore natural function and balance.*

Care Is Discipline

The National Weight Control Registry (NWCR) established by Rena Wing, Ph.D. and James Hill, Ph.D. in 1993 has added to our understanding of weight loss maintenance. The registry has information on 3000 people who lost 30 to 100 pounds and maintained a stable weight for at least one year.

How did they do it?

Statistics show the people were highly disciplined about keeping food diaries, counting calories and recording their weight. They scheduled their exercise on their calendars and followed through with discipline. Also, people in the registry burned up about 2700 calories a week in physical activity like walking one mile a day for a weekly sum of five miles.

Moreover, people developed a new mind set about food. They didn't struggle over the salad or the French fries and burger. They simply put the fries and burger out of their mind, in effect, limiting their choices.

> *My personal experience is to focus on my body size and shape rather than weight.*

Therefore I insist that my patients measure the circumference of the neck, chest, upper arms, upper thighs, waist, and buttocks. Put these numbers away at the beginning of the journey. Then re-measure every month to keep track of your progress. This system reinforces your success without your constant worry over it because whatever you are doing, it is part of your lifestyle and you are going to stay with it! Patients could *monitor their loss simply by their belts or the clothes being looser, and they have the pleasure of buying smaller and smaller clothe sizes.*

DOCTOR TAI'S IMPORTANT TIP

Describe in writing what your care culture would be for yourself. Design your care program to include what food you prefer, your serving size and exercises for a week. Then choose a protein breakfast menu for week one. Share your plan with a partner or friend so you have someone with whom you can be accountable and discuss the progress being made.

Chapter Five

EXCITED TO DEATH

 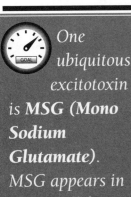

*One ubiquitous excitotoxin is **MSG (Mono Sodium Glutamate)**. MSG appears in almost all fast or processed foods, snack foods such as chips and crackers, plus seasoning mixtures and flavoring sauces. They are hidden in foods as well under the names of hydrolyzed yeast, yeast extract, soy extract and protein isolate. They are further disguised as "secret" ingredients or proprietary recipes served in restaurants.*

Excito-what?

Most of us would agree that the American media and advertising has sold us all on the joys of eating and stuffing our faces with addictive, high calorie food that have no nutritional value. Mmmm…but doesn't it taste good?

Those tasty little molecules that make our mouths salivate; our brains gyrate and our bodies gain weight are called excitotoxins. Or, they are better described as taste enhancers that are poisons, which we put into our phenomenal human forms.

Aspartame is the most well known excitotoxin because the FDA approved this substance as a sugar substitute in 1981. Now, it is found in diet drinks, foods, and in artificial sweeteners like Equal and NutraSweet. Aspartame gets a lot of press for good reason: FDA approved it, yet research clearly shows the toxic effects of the substance.

Even though these substances do make bland foods tasty by stimulating the brain's pleasure centers, you will do best by avoiding them altogether. *Research in China showed that those who ate the* most MSG were three times as likely to be overweight. Aspartame may cause weight gain even though a person has lower caloric intake.

Ignorance Is Bliss

Louisa, who recently became pregnant, is a customer service counselor who sits all day at her desk and computer, talking to customers on the phone. Her aspartame addiction started easily enough, just one-diet soda in the morning to get her started. She stopped drinking coffee because of her pregnancy. On her lunch break, however, she had another diet soda, the kind with caffeine in it for a midday pick-me-up. By two in the afternoon, she could see how edgy and restless she was. Thinking she was just tired from the pregnancy, Louisa had another diet soda at 3 pm and another at 4 pm. She did feel more upbeat although her irritation and restlessness increased.

Aspartame and MSG cause identical adverse reactions in people who are sensitive to them. Both have been shown to kill brain cells and cause subsequent endocrine disorders in laboratory animals.

Louisa decided to talk to her Supervisor and coach about cutting back on her hours. Her coach had recently returned from maternity leave herself. After Louisa stated her fatigue, hunger for coffee, her new diet of snack foods and drinks at her desk, her coach, Krista, raised her hand to stop her.

DOCTOR TAI'S IMPORTANT TIP

What sweeteners are safe to use? Try Stevia because it is derived from the Stevia bush, which grows wild in the rain forests. Used as a sweetener and for medicinal purposes by natives, it is suitable for diabetics in improving glucose tolerance and aids your body in lowering blood pressure.

Krista said, "Louisa, let me stop you there. I went through exactly the same thing you are experiencing, and you need some new information to make better choices. My mom is a nutritionist and she set me straight on foods and drinks.

Krista continued, "First, you say you want no caffeine, so that means no coffee or the soft drinks you are having, both of which have caffeine. The reason for your growing agitation is an ingredient called aspartame in the sodas. Every soft drink you have adds to your chances of having diabetes. Here is what I drink."

Krista pulled open a desk drawer to reveal an array of herbal teas and small bottles of water, which she refilled from the jugs of spring water in the employee lounge.

"See," Krista continued, "I choose from a variety of teas. I like green tea a lot. So, if your goals are to be healthy, have a healthy baby, and keep up the hours, then let's work out your lunch breaks, snack breaks, and exercise on a twenty minute cycle, even if you stretch or walk around the building. You can have a healthy routine here at the office, and I'll support you in it one hundred per cent. Mostly you need to educate yourself about what goes into your mouth. After all, there are two of you now!"

Aspartame

Aspartame has three substances. Two are amino acids and the third is methanol, also known as wood alcohol, a neurotoxin.

The two amino acids are vital to normal brain function and yet, they become toxic in excess.

The media convinced most people to drink diet sodas for their health rather than sugar-laden drinks. We believed and poured it down, sometimes enough to cause severe difficulties like in the following examples:

• A mom calls because she thinks her eight-year-old son is showing symptoms of bipolar disorder in that he flies and then falls in his moods. A review of his dietary habits showed that the boy drank up to eight diet sodas a day.

• A graduate student earned his doctorate in psychology and started his first job in a private mental health clinic. Being with clients seven hours a day wearied him, and he started drinking more coffee plus diet soft drinks throughout the day. He noticed two specific behavioral changes. The first was that he became more agitated. The second was he noticed negative thought spirals about his clients, such as they were neurotic addicts, immature emotionally… By the end of his workday, he noticed that he was physically exhausted.

• A fifteen-year-old local baseball star started having seizures during training. He drank more and more sodas with aspartame in the heat of the day, trying to restore energy. Instead, he was causing neuronal firing.

Brain Poisons

In his article, "Aspartame Disease: an FDA Approved Epidemic," H.J. Roberts, MD, writes, "Diet products, which contain the chemical sweetener aspartame have multiple neurotoxic, metabolic, allergenic, fetal and carcinogenic effects."[8] Dr. Roberts, Director of the Palm Beach Institute for Medical Research, coined the term "Aspartame Disease" because he has researched 1200 aspartame reactors in his database, and published in his book Aspartame Disease: *an Ignored Epidemic* (Sunshine Sentinel Press, 2001). The specific reactors included problems with eyes, ears, heart, skin allergies, gastrointestinal, muscular, and endocrine disorders plus specific symptoms of neurological, psychiatric, and kidney issues. Of course, the list includes Weight Disorders!

 Excitotoxin's effect on brain cells is to "excite them to death." They are present in most all processed

---

[8] http://articles.mercola.com/sites/articles/archive/2004/01/07/aspartame-disease-part-two.aspx

57

> *"I have tried to show the reader that there is a strong connection between dietary and endogenous excitotoxin excess and neurological dysfunction and disease. As our knowledge of the pathophysiology and biochemistry of the neurodegenerative diseases increases, the connection to excitotoxicity has become stronger."*

foods in forms like natural flavoring, spices, or textured protein extract. The more notable excitotoxin is MSG-Monosodium Glutamate.

Russell Blaylock, MD, neurologist, researcher and author of the book *Excitotoxins: The Taste That Kills* (Health Press, 1997) wrote,

High Fructose Corn Syrup

Another deadly excitotoxin is high fructose corn syrup. This is made by treating corn with different enzymes to extract the sugar glucose, convert it to fructose, and produce an exceptionally sweet taste. By 2001, corn sweeteners became the top sweetener because of lower production costs. The public's consumption went *from zero in 1966 to 62 pounds per person in 2001*. Here is how it affects the body:

- Fructose does not stimulate insulin production.
- Fructose does not increase leptin production.
- We need adequate insulin and leptin production to help the body turn off appetite.
- Thus excess fructose with excess calories is a huge contributor to obesity.

Rod Gustafson, columnist for *Parenting and the Media* (parentstv.org) summarized research by a school nurse on obesity in American adolescents and found that soft drinks made up "a significant portion of the calorie intake in an average teen's day." Gustafson goes on to explain that the media war between the two biggest soft drink advertisers flood adolescents' brains with images of athletes and models guzzling the liquid gold filled with high calorie high glycemic corn syrup fructose.

Paradoxical Images

Media images that make women feel fat even when they are perfectly healthy are the topics of shows like ABC's *The View*. The American public's distorted images of food and fashion have been called "schizophrenic." Dinners, lunches, business and socializing are all invested in shared food and fun, soothing food bits and tantalizing appetizers. The paradoxical message, however, is stay thin, fashionable, lovely, agile and muscular while maintaining those social circles and hearty appetites.

We can hold the image of the skinny beauty or muscle man in our minds as our goals. Or we can feel intimidated and stick to sweatshirt and oversize tee shirts as comfort clothes that hide our bodies. The only way we personally will survive the Hollywood influence is to have a strong self-image and take daily steps to good health like eating and exercising appropriately.

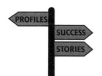

Chard's Story

During the eight-week bauhinia trial, Chard lost four pounds. "I did not drop a lot of weight, but I lost a considerable amount in inches," he said, and he was referring to three inches from his waist and from his hips, which were part of the measurements of the study. Chard added, "But I also lost from my chest and arms. The Thin Factors is making a huge impact in my life. Every day, people tell me they see a difference in my appearance. Friends I have not seen in a while ask me how I have dropped the inches. I was able to get back to my ideal size and weight."

Surveys show that the gap is widening between self-perceived weight and self-reported weight. Women think of themselves as overweight and men under-estimate their weight. None of us will work as hard at dieting or exercise as the brawny and the beautiful in media, but we have great options for looking good and being healthy. In section four, you'll find the **most practical and successful program for your Vitality and Wellness.**

Consider the words of Mohandas Gandhi:

"Our thoughts become our words as they become our beliefs; our beliefs become our actions as they become our habits. Our habits become our values as our values become our destiny."

We have the ability to overcome the Hollywood influence! Let's do it!

Chapter Six

STRESS-FULL LIVING

The time to relax is when you don't have time for it.
Author Unknown

A Hidden, Powerful Player in the Weight Game

Many patients have said to me that they hear so much about stress, they could scream. Yet, when moving through days of busy-ness and business, the word stress is on no one's mind. Our attention is focused on managing the events around us.

Think of Stress, then, as circumstances that stretch you to the edge or beyond coping abilities. They could be major events or minor events in any given day.

> *The key is your emotional response to those events. Stress is really more about our capacity to handle change than it is about whether that change makes us feel good or bad.*

So the emotional reactions to stress that occur on biochemical levels have significant effects and are often unnoticed by us. Stress is quiet, creating small ripples and reactions that accrue over time inside our bodies. Then one day, we suddenly notice that we are not well or inflammation has flared up in a joint or in the colon, and stress has deposited in the form of fat globules inflating our waist.

Each time we have a startle response, an anger reaction or an irritating day, the body gives us a *shot of adrenaline*, which activates the stress hormone, **cortisol**. If you rest or slow down from startle or agitation, then the body relaxes, and you recover quickly.

The Chronic Culprit

When you don't slow down or relax, chronic stress is the culprit. Perhaps you get up late, hurry to and through work, skip a meal, skip your walk, and remain generally irritated or agitated. At the end of your day, you have a beer or three. If that is your normal day, then you are killing yourself because the slow-down and recovery time never happens. Bodies can be stressed or even should be stressed because that is part of normal living, even make it through the toughest times, but they need to recover as a protective measure.

☞ *The extent of damage due to stress is dependent directly on the **intensity** and the **duration** of the stress event and ultimate immediate **recovery**.*

Stress Link to Obesity

The journal *Nature*[9] reported the results of a study by Georgetown University's Department of Physiology and Biophysics.

☞*Research demonstrated that a neuropeptide Y (NY), a stress molecule, unlocks Y2 receptors in fat cells. Researchers also showed that blocking that Y2 switch prevents fat accumulation and shrink fat deposits.*

Researchers subjected mice to *chronic stress*, and then gave them the equivalent of a human junk food diet...*high fat and high sugar.* After two weeks, the mice that were stressed and ate the junk food diet gained significant weight with *two times more belly fat than their non-stressed* counterparts. Moreover, those mice gained the toxic fat deposited around the belly that creates the chemical signals associated with illness. We discuss these chemical signals thoroughly in the next section on fat.

In summary, *a stressed body releases a molecule called neuropeptide Y (NPY), which unlocks Y2 receptors in fat cells,*

---

[9] Kuo, Lydia E. et al. "Corrigenda: Neuropeptide Y acts directly in the periphery on fat tissue and mediates stress-induced obesity and metabolic syndrome." Nature Medicine (09-01-07

and then fat cells grow in size and number. In addition, NPY contributes to other stress-related problems that lower immune system strength, leading to frequent bouts of cold and illnesses.

DOCTOR TAI'S IMPORTANT TIP

Taking a stress break is as easy as walking around your office or sitting in your chair and practicing brief strategies, the effect of which are to relax and calm. Visualizing your favorite vacation scene and breathing consciously for several moments feels like you just returned from that week off. Close your eyes and imagine.... You are walking on a pristine white sandy beach in Hawaii or Fiji or at the snowy Rocky mountain ski trails... Walk the beach; ski down the soft powder and feel the wind. Breathe in the fresh air.

Relax... relax...

Spend the next five minutes breathing in through your nose and exhaling through your mouth while you enjoy the scenery and sunshine.

Cortisol Effects

One of the main effects of stress, then, is increasing cortisol levels, which causes weight gain by increasing the amount of unhealthy fat. Our bodies store fat under the skin (subcutaneous) and internally around organs like our hearts and livers. The internal fat is visceral, from viscera, meaning internal organs. It is also called the **Omentum**. Health practitioners consider the visceral fat as unhealthy.

Why? Too much visceral fat is one symptom of the larger cluster called **Metabolic X Syndrome**, which is discussed in depth in later chapters. If you have increased visceral fat, most likely you have problems with all four hormones: *Thyroid, cortisol, leptin and insulin.*

This discussion of stress and obesity helps us understand that overweight conditions and obesity are not caused by psychological factors such as weak will power, poor focus or laziness. Psychology does contribute, but the more we view the brain and body as a closed-loop system of stimulus-response, we gain strength in how to make better lifestyle choices.

The chart below indicates research results and how some patients who fit in those stress categories chose different lifestyle strategies for the sake of their health.

RESEARCH CONCLUSIONS	LIFESTYLE STRATEGIES
Charles P. Vega, MD, Associate Professor, Department of Family Medicine, University of California, Irvine, reports that job stress is a major factor that contributes to obesity."[10] From a study of 10, 308 civil servants (ages 35-55), men suffered the job stress through obesity more than women.	Lou gained weight when he was laid off and switched to a new job. He was on his feet all day and chose to bounce on a mini-trampoline to keep energized and exercised. On the other hand, Christopher worked at a desk and computer all day at a sales office. Breaks were scheduled every forty minutes, and he utilized the time for yogic stretching instead of snacking or drinking more coffee like his cohorts.
In a survey of more than 1,800 people last year, the American Psychological Association reports 43 percent of respondents admitted to overeating or to eating unhealthy foods in response to stress during the previous month. And women were more apt to do it than men.	Jane, a high-powered attorney who worked long hours, started a morning meditation group for the workers who arrived early or were interested in stress management. Lynn changed her snacking at her desk routines to drinking tea. She also joined a women's support group, which helped her refocus her priorities and habits.

[10] http://www.mentalhelp.net/poc/view_doc.php?type=weblog&id=294&wlid=5&cn=117

Sleeping for less than six hours a night can cause cortisol levels to rise by fifty percent.	Jake, at age fifteen, was gaining weight. He rarely slept because of his intense focus on Xbox and gaming. When his parents noticed depression creeping in, they sat in conversation. Jake and his parents developed a contract holding Jake accountable for so many hours of workout at their local fitness center.

Belly Size Matters

A groundbreaking new study focused on whether size really matters. As more men and women become overweight, the more we customize ourselves to a new, larger norm. This is not healthy.

Boston researchers completed a large study on women, obesity, and fitness.[4] They tracked for ten years the overall health profiles of 39,000 women, with an average age of 54. Thirty-four percent exercised regularly, 31 percent were overweight, and 18 percent were obese. None showed signs of heart disease, diabetes, or cancer at the start of the study.[11]

By the end of the study, they found that with regular exercise, heart disease rates were still a lot higher even for women with "a little extra padding." The risk

[11] Weinstein et al. "The joint effects of physical activity and body mass index on coronary heart disease risk in women." Archives of Internal Medicine. 168:884-890.

was 54 percent higher for this group and 87 percent higher for active but obese women. **Size does matter.**

The **amount of belly fat** also matters. *The New England Journal of Medicine* (November 12, 2008) reports the effects of following 360,000 Europeans in a long-term health study.

One finding was that people with the most belly fat doubled their risk of dying prematurely compared to people with the least belly fat. Death risk increased with weight circumference despite normal weight.[12]

[12] Pischon, T. The New England Journal of Medicine, (11-12-08) Vol. 359: pp 2105-2120.

Belly Fat is mostly white adipose tissue called Omentum which is known to produce **adipokinins**, spewing these highly inflammatory compounds all over the body elevating blood **C-reactive protein, CRP**, the inflammation marker leading to arthritis, lower immunity, cancer and heart disease. As if this not enough, these **excess fat cells makes extra estrogen**, a specific female hormone that significantly increases incidence of breast tumors. For men, estrogen decidedly makes them more feminine and lowers libido. There also appears to be direct correlation between the amount of belly fat and the fat around your heart. So that big belly fat can literally tell you that you maybe choking your heart to death with the fat surrounding it.

So how do you make your size the right size if you tend to be overweight?

What's Up Ahead!

This chapter discussed chronic stress and the relationship of stress to fat and concluded that belly fat is unhealthy. In the next section…

• First, I'll give you the skinny on fat. If you understand how you make fat and what habits lead to fat, then you can change what doesn't work.

• Then we'll review the science of appetite and the hormones that play roles in the crucial balance for health.

The hormonal imbalances of overweight, obesity and subsequent inflammatory conditions are covered in detail. Then we'll return to how science has done its part of completing studies of Bauhinia that encourage this herb's cleansing, detoxing, and rejuvenating the metabolism and the participation in our return to awesome health.

Part III

FAT HAS A LIFE
OF ITS OWN

Chapter Seven

WHY ARE WE TOPPING OUT AND HANGING OVER?

Love That Cellulite!

Since obesity is at epidemic proportions, let me educate you on some facts about the fat cells and what kinds of fat we have.

- *First, fat is the only tissue in our bodies that has unlimited growth potential throughout your entire life.*

- *Secondly, fat cells vary by type, location and function. We've learned the two locations are under the skin (subcutaneous) and inside the body around internal organs (visceral).*

- *Thirdly, fat functions include regulation of hormone production, heat generation, metabolism and body weight.*

- *Finally, fat cells are called **adipocytes** (a-depe-sits), and there are two types: **BAT** refers to brown adipose tissue and **WAT** refers to white adipose tissue…thus brown fat and white fat are quite different.*

BAT - What bears and babies have in common is brown adipose tissue (BAT) or brown fat. Brown fat burns energy to generate heat. Newborns have brown fat to regulate their body temperature and bears in hibernation through the winter stay normalized. Brown fat is so named because of its characteristic brown color from its greater blood supply in between the fat cells.

Researchers found that brown fat is closely associated with muscle, burns calories and releases energy. In short, BAT has a strong **thermogenic effect.**

The brain, nerves, and stress hormones, such as epinephrine and norepinephrine, control BAT. A special receptor, called **B-3**, for these stress hormones is found only in BAT. Stimulation of ***the B-3 receptor boosts metabolism by increasing heat production and fat breakdown.*** We want this!

> *Being overweight means that BAT does **not** produce adequate amount of thermogenins, the protein that produces heat. So overweight, which is to say our hormones are out of balance, equals slower metabolism from lower thyroid level, lower heat production from thyroid receptor resistance, therefore much lower resting calorie expenditure, resulting in more difficulty with weight loss. Hormonal imbalance equates to increased appetite, slower metabolism, fat deposited in the belly and omentum, **inside** muscles and organs.*

WAT – White adipose tissue, WAT for short, is all over our bodies, mostly under our skin. Most women would recognize this as *cellulite*. Our tissues store excess energy in the form of fat cells.

*White adipose tissue produces hormones like **leptin** (regulates fat storage), **adiponectin** (regulates lipids and glucose), **adipokinins** (inflammation igniters) and **resistin** (contributes to insulin resistance).*

Mostly WAT accumulates in our bellies (Omentum) and make our enormous waist. All of this is caused by our bio-hormone imbalances, the excess sugar in our blood. After the big meal, the sugar has no place to go, so the body stores it for future use as fat around your waist and belly.

> *So white fat stores energy, brown fat releases energy.*
> *Remember this word—**thermogenesis**—the key to your*
> *metabolism, which the brain and body chemical processes that*
> *maintain life. When you exercise, you start your engine and*
> *increase your metabolism. When you increase speed, distance,*
> *energy and effort, you rev up the engine, heating up your body*
> *and making it work harder. That thermogenic effect burns fat.*

Lower body temperature means a lower metabolism, and you'll find exercises in later chapters for warming up slowly and gaining strength and endurance.

When it comes to fat storage, we describe men and women as having the shape of an apple or a pear. Women generally gain white fat around the buttocks and thighs, appearing pear-shaped, this maybe a reflection of hormone **progesterone**. Men gain it mostly around the abdomen, presenting an apple-like profile, maybe a influence of imbalance from testosterone and **estrogen**.

Because of our fat profiles, most people think that fat sets up house in a body part, like the thighs or the abdomen, and starts hoarding more fat cells. But this is not the case.

Listen To Your Fat!

Sometimes I imagine a conversation between white adipose tissue lamenting that the woman hates her body and her fat. Eavesdrop on this conversation between WAT and its therapist named Doc.

"Doc," says WAT, "she doesn't understand me."

"Really?"

"No, no she doesn't. She complains about me constantly, always telling her friend that she has to fight me! Doc, why does she want to fight with me?"

"Why do you think?"

"Well, doesn't she know that I'm just doing my job? I store

fat. She may need me in the future. I help her if she ever faces starvation!"

"Yes, you do! It sounds like she can only see the outside, cottage-cheese skin, not the loving fat inside who is doing its job, and all for her survival!"

"And there's more, she thinks I suddenly appeared as a beach ball in her belly. That's just not true. She doesn't know my nature. Fat develops in layers, slowly growing like a onion, working hard to plump each fat cell bigger and fatter."

"I didn't know that."

"Yes, it's true. I will come off layer by layer and shrink each fat cell. So what does she do? She bends me on an AB machine, ten minutes every day. She's even threatening to increase the time to 30 minutes daily. She believes so desperately that I'll just go away, she bought a second machine. I am scared of what desperate measure she is thinking next …Surgical Liposuction?

You know, Doc, I just don't disappear like magic from her belly or bottom. I come off like onion layers from within the whole body as each fat cell shrink to its original birth size."

"I can see that you would like her to save her money on machines and talk with you to learn more about you."

"Yes, Doc! That would help! She's even considering going on one of those fad diets that completely cuts out dietary fat, like olive oil and Omega 3, a vital source of energy and health. What can I do?"

DOCTOR TAI'S IMPORTANT TIP

*Understand how your body works. Fat stores, called omentum, are around internal organs and under skin. Exercise supports weight loss subcutaneously. Dieting results in more fat loss viscerally or **omentum**, and you may not immediately notice any radical difference in your appearance, but it is there and its benefits are cumulative.*

Stay committed to your health goals anyway. Some people like overworked athletic women or anorexic persons have too little body fat, and this causes physiological complications, like the cessation of menses. Too much body fat is also harmful. For men whose fat index is over 25% and women's over 30%, there is a dramatic correlation of excessive body fat with higher frequency of illness and disease, like hypertension, diabetes, cancer and heart problems.

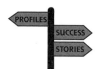

PROFILES SUCCESS STORIES

Jim's Story

Jim had never been on a diet. He spent his 56 years in the small town of Thomaston, Georgia where he worked hard at a textile factory and hunted and fished on weekends. With all of these physical demands, going to the gym seemed beside the point, as did saying no to one more biscuit or helping of gravy.

An authentic Southern "good ole boy," who married his high school sweetheart and gorged happily on her home coming for forty years, Jim stood six feet tall, but his weight topped out at 316 pounds. Jim said in his country drawl, "I figured I'd just tote whatever weight I had as long as my friends could carry me to the grave when the time came. I honestly didn't realize that I'd gotten that big and out of shape." But he had.

Jim suffered from cardiovascular problems, and his knee-replacement surgery reduced his activity level even more. He was an unlikely dieter who needed help. When his doctor approached him about participating in the bauhinia clinical trials for weight loss, he said, "Why not?"

Before each meal, Jim drank one glass of water mixed with five milliliters of an extract (2 Gelcaps) from the leaves of Bauhinia. The supplement immediately decreased his appetite. **"I noticed that I didn't need as much food to fill me up. I generally felt better all the way around."**

When attending church services, Jim wore a suit that he hadn't fit into for five years. The preacher gave a double take, and friends in the congregation cheered him on. Jim 12-year-old grandson patted him on the belly and said, Pawpaw, your belly used to be way out there, and now it is way back here. Jim explained, "I didn't know my grandson had noticed, but my belly must have been bad if he was following my weight loss."

In one month, Jim dropped 14 pounds. He continued with the trials for another four weeks and lost an additional 9 pounds, for a **total of 23 whopping pounds**. *His fifty-eight inch waist shrank by* **four inches**. *In total, Jim's weight at the end of the 60 day clinical study using the* **The Thin Factors** *was 280 pounds.*

Chapter Eight

Hormones Regulate
the Rhythms

The Communication System

Our entire physical structure survives through a delicate system of communication through **hormones, the messengers**. *Natural Hormones (not synthetic) are significant players in your best health and in the quality of your life. They regulate metabolism,* and hormone miscommunication can influence the onset of disease, as later chapters will reveal.

Let's understand how hormones work. These chemical messengers that endocrine glands produce and secrete into the bloodstream cause actions at a distant location in the body. In essence, they coordinate the body's functions through their communication—ongoing signals to and from the brain. One example of their complexity is that *nineteen hormones manage appetite and weight alone.*

Old & Fat
The older you get,
the fewer active leptin receptors you have in your hypothalamus. The less sensitive your satiety signals are, the more prone

to munching you will be. Satiety malfunction causes weight gain.
At the center of your brain, the hypothalamus control appetite and thirst. Craving starts in your brain!

Every organ or tissue in the body can act like a gland to make hormones. Some hormones are made from cholesterol, while others are made from protein. For example, **fat cells make protein hormones called leptin and adiponectin, which are keys to our appetite and weight health.**

Once a gland sends a hormone to the nerves, liver, heart kidneys…the hormone find its *target, a receptor on a cell. Like a key slipping into a lock, the hormone and receptor merge, and chemical action ensues.* For example,

- A thyroid hormone finds its receptor on the heart, which then beats stronger, overcoming heart enlargement (ventricular hypertrophy).

- Thyroid sends a hormone to a receptor on the intestines, and they move faster, overcoming chronic constipation.

- Leptin receptors, while all over the body, have a main location is the appetite control center of the brain, the hypothalamus.

• Brains receptors can shut down appetite and speed up metabolism.

Hormones cycle at peaks and lows, according to our body rhythms. Cortisol, testosterone and glucagon peak in the morning. Leptin and growth hormone, for example, peak in the middle of the night. Eating in the middle of the night (between 2am and 4am) can disrupt hormonal balance and lead to severe weight gain.

Four Hormonal Groups

Body communication through hormones is structured according to the hormone's functions. They are interactive, of course, among the four functional groups of hormones: sexuality, metabolism, stress, and regulatory.

In my book, **8 Powerful Secrets to Anti-Aging**, I describe in detail the functions of hormones as they affect our health, sexuality and metabolism.

DOCTOR TAI'S IMPORTANT TIP

Dr. T. Villarreal revealed the effects of DHEA on abdominal fat in elderly men and woman. He found DHEA supplements reduce visceral fat, so called "abdominal fat" significantly. (JAMA, Nov. 2004).

Together, DHEA and pregnenolone are by far the most abundant and pre-eminent hormones because they actually precede the other hormones.

Master Hormones – Pregnenolone and DHEA control the brain's memory functions; and DHEA is a powerful natural hormone of activity and antiAging.

Sex hormones – The primary sex hormones are estrogen, testosterone, and progesterone. Sex hormones define gender and regulate reproduction. Estrogen also influences brain communications, moods and deposits fat on the butt and thighs. Testosterone builds muscles in the deposit of fat around the belly and interacts with estrogen in influencing emotionality.

Although men and women both have estrogen and androgen hormones, they differ vastly between genders. Female ovaries produce estrogens and progesterone to stimulate the growth of sex organs, breasts and also regulate menses. Male testes produce androgens and regulate the sex drive, sculpting the body muscle and emotional confidence.

*When women enter **menopause**, they gain excess weight around the waist and hips. Men also experience a similar midlife pause called **andropause** in which they experience an increase of estrogen in the form of higher estrone and estradiol. These two hormones increase fat deposits around the waist and hips, feminizing the men's bodies, even increasing fat deposits around the chest into small breast formation called gynecomastia.*

Metabolic hormones – Metabolism means the chemical processes that regulate the rate of energy expenditure and functions of our vital organs that give us life. The hormones of the thyroid, insulin and growth hormone regulate our physiology such as how we convert food to fuel, burn calories, store fat, and many of the digestive processes we have discussed in this book.

Disturbance in the balance of metabolic hormones in men and women results in lowering our resting metabolic burn rate...leading to less burned calories per day to maintain bodily functions and lower thermogenic heat production.

Remember that we need thermogenesis to be at a good level to burn off the calories and keep our active vitality.

As we age, our decrease in burned calories becomes obvious. We slow down our daily activity, feel colder and lose muscle tone. *This metabolic downturn also is present after we try a crash diet, become ill, or develop nutritional deficiencies like missing protein-amino acids, vitamins, and micro-minerals like iodine, zinc and selenium.*

Our options are to exercise and increase the metabolism or reduce calorie intake. In the absence of increased exercise, you must reduce caloric intake or the excess calories (above the function of daily body maintenance) will turn into fat cells and weight gain that averages into a half pound a month, or 5 pounds a year. That is 50 pounds in 10 years. Trust me, you don't want the additional weight or the health problems it brings you.

DOCTOR TAI'S IMPORTANT TIP

Manage all hormonal imbalances. You can't always control your hormone levels. When ghrelin levels overcome leptin, and you feel hungry, develop ahead of time a list of emergency foods to satisfy you when cravings set in. Try V8 juice, a handful of nuts, cut up vegetables or natural yogurt with sugar free fruit, or ice tea.

Circadian hormones – When we travel and move around the globe or shift time zones and altitudes, hormones like melatonin and parathyroid keep our bodies regulated within the environments.

You will gain one to two pounds in a week while traveling through 4 or more time zones. To not gain weight, you must make your adjustments quickly and decisively. *Getting plenty of sleep.* Sunlight exposure is critical to time adjustment. Also, *melatonin supplementation at night* can help to facilitate the transition without excessive food cravings, hunger and eating at odd hours.

Take advantage of your body's own set weight by making small corrections of dietary caloric intake right away. Then you will shed any excess weight from your travels within ten days. The reason you must act immediately to shed the weight is that your body readjusts your *set weight to higher poundage.*

Stress hormones – We've already mentioned stress hormones like cortisol, epinephrine, and norepinephrine, which the brain and adrenal glands produce when we go on alert or into high gear. Stress hormones have benefits to mobilize sugar for immediate conversion to energy.

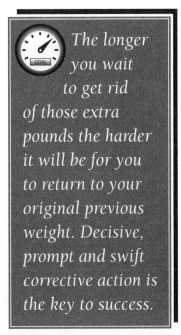

The longer you wait to get rid of those extra pounds the harder it will be for you to return to your original previous weight. Decisive, prompt and swift corrective action is the key to success.

Stress hormones like cortisol and adrenaline are all glucose mobilizers. In other words they cause an immediate rise in blood sugars and move the liver to manufacture more sugars all in the name of survival. Yes, Survival! The body thinks that you are going to use the extra sugar as immediate energy to make an emergency escape from a dangerous lion.

Your body doesn't know that you are sitting comfortably in your gas guzzling, four-wheel-drive, oversized SUV, and you were stressed because the traffic isn't moving as fast as you want. Nope, your body doesn't know the nature of your stress episode. Rather, your body just knows you are having one!

So the enormous extra sugar overload isn't being used for anything while your body just sits there, waiting for you to run five miles as fast as you can to secure your survival.

So the body waits….and waits. Nothing happens. A befuddled body just deposits bigger, plumper fat cells right on your waist, getting ready to be used in the next emergency survival episode.

That is how recurrent consistent stress turns into frequent deposits of fat around your waist **every time you get mad** at the grocery clerk, miss a deadline or have one of those difficult conversations with your boss or spouse. **You just keep depositing more layers of fat!**

Even worse evidence-based science shows that excess chronic cortisol causes muscle waste and loss of muscle mass, leaving you weak with lower metabolic rate because of loss of energy burn from lack of muscle.[13]

DOCTOR TAI'S IMPORTANT TIP

Stress Busters By Temperament Types

The way you handle stress may be tied directly into your temperament or the type of personality you were born with. Generally, each person falls into one category and usually two.

Doer: *For example, you may be a doer and get upset if your activities are interrupted, hindered or left unfinished. You work hard, even persevering through fatigue. Manage your stress using your strength of being a doer. What exercise can you do while you sit it traffic? Deep breathing and isometrics! Strategize or review your game plan? Dictate your creativity for later transcription? Can you rise earlier and get to the office before traffic? Will you build stressor breaks into your daily schedule so you can focus better and produce more?*

Learner: *Since you love to learn, choose MP3 files you can download to an Ipod when you drive. Listen to audio books. Schedule your exercise routine around a quiet walk or contemplation if you need to review information. When*

---

[13] Kaplan,S. et al. "Effects of cortisol on amino acid in skeletal muscle and plasma," Endocrinology 72(1963):267

you get mentally overwhelmed, then switch to easy-listening music or seek silent meditation to calm your mind.

Harmonizer: *Since you seek harmony and need an easy-going flow in life, you have to take extra care to structure your time and environment to accommodate your stress. Your stress revolves around doing too much, helping others non-stop, always being compliant. Your gift is bringing practical solutions to people and you can do this for your stress also. Since you don't always plan ahead, then make your daily resilience builders about taking the right balance of vitamins, minerals, antioxidants, and herbal rejuvenators (see www.healthsecretsusa.com), walking every morning, taking a mid-morning tai chi break, listening to enjoyable music as you drive.*

Expresser: *As a highly intuitive people-person, you can easily lose track of time, burn out, and over react. Your stress busters involve moving excess energy out of your body... try a treadmill, dancing, writing in a diary, yogic stretching. As you drive, dictate your creativity into a tape recorder for later transcription. Listen to your body before you get burned out...meaning don't have the second helping or the piece of key lime pie. Because you lose track of time, you absolutely must clock yourself with reminders from your PDA, turn your clock back by fifteen minutes so you'll be ahead of yourself, do your exercise every day at the same time with no excuses, and limit telephone calls to a specific time frame. Soft and upbeat music is your listening background soothes your stressors.*

Hormones Imbalances

Hormone imbalances can cause communication problems with tissues. *In a normal functioning body, when a hormone, the key, inserts in a cell's receptor, a special communication with a set of instructions is taking place; normal biochemistry stays in good working order. If the hormone keys cannot enter the cell receptor lock, the communication goes haywire. The receptor and the cells are starving for the hormone, a condition called* **Receptor Resistance or Receptor Insensitivity**. Your body suffers from hormone deficiency, even though there is often no shortage of blood circulating the hormone.

The miscommunication causes further problems. The gland continues to be told to produce more hormones in desperation to make good on the receptors lack of satisfaction, which keep sending SOS signals to the brain that the cells and tissues are starving for the hormone.

Even when you are suffering from all the classical signs and symptoms of hormone deficiency, *your doctor continues to insist that the blood test shows you have plenty of hormones.* Therefore, nothing is wrong with you, so either you are getting old or just plain crazy. Most likely, your doctor says, *"I know the problem. You must be depressed. What you really need is a strong dose of antidepressants. Here's your prescription, and I'll see you in six months. Please don't call me; I'll call you. Have a great day!"*

Of course, when you read the fine print of antidepressants' side effects, it explains that this will lead to further weight gain and hormonal deficiencies. For those of us who are out of shape and overweight, our bodies have communication problems. Let's see how this affects the metabolic hormones, eating and appetite.

Chapter Nine

THE SCIENCE OF APPETITE

The tongue is the body's most powerful muscle, with papillae that detect the chemicals in foods and signal tastes. There are approximately 10,000 taste buds in an average person. People restore new taste buds every three to ten days, but the restoration rate become slower as people get older. Elderly people may have only 5,000 taste buds.

Good Intentions!

Lindsey, a mom of three in sunny Florida, had her children within a five-year time span and exercised for the first year after her last child's birth. She felt good during that year, and as the children grew into preschool age, she lost track of her time and her health. All her good intentions disappeared over five years in which she gained enough weight to be classified as mildly obese. Her blood sugar levels started to rise, making her a prime candidate for diabetes type 2.

Lindsey's mother has been in professional real estate for thirty years and thrived in the joy of networking and sales. When she entered menopause she exercised more and maintained a simple diet of whole grains, vegetables and proteins. Yet, she started adding a pound or two over time, all in the abdomen. She was embarrassed by her weight and did not understand what had changed within her despite a healthy diet, exercise three times a week, and an active lifestyle.

Each person's story involved good intentions, yet without satisfactory results, because they were not educated as to the relationship between the act of eating, the chemistry of appetite and how the body controls weight. In fact, scientists are still learning right now about new aspects of the 45 hormones that contribute to appetite.

Out of Control Appetites

In our evolution, the appetite driver serves our survival as a species. The appetite control system registers when we have had enough to eat, tells us when to stop, or tells us when we are hungry.

The complex dance of hormonal communications involves the brain, the nervous system, metabolic hormones, special fat cells and the immune system. I've explained how the systems of stressors, fats, and hormones communicate in previous chapters.

Out of control hormones tell us to eat when we don't need to and lead to significant health risks. More importantly, it can happen to a toddler, child or adult, of any ethnicity or environment. The **Globesity** epidemic affects all of us now. In all honesty, scientists are finding out just how little we know.

For example, **forty known receptor sites in the brain play a role in feeling hungry or being full, and the estimate is that there could be 100 more.**

> ## Food Fights in the Brain
>
> • *The satiety center is controlled by CART (Cocaine, Amphetamine, Regulatory and Transcript).*
>
> • *CART stimulates the hypothalamus to increase metabolism, reduce appetite, and increases insulin to raise energy to muscle cells and reduce fat.*
>
> • *NPY (Neuropeptide Y) affects the hypothalamus by decreasing metabolism and increasing appetite.*
>
> • *Higher levels of leptin from FAT cells and intestines lower appetite and eating when receptors are functioning normally.*
>
> • *Empty stomachs increase ghrelin, making you hungry and promoting eating.*

Metabolic hormones like insulin, thyroid, growth hormone, testosterone, estrogen and many others influence the appetite control system. Hormones coordinate and regulate all aspects of appetite and satiety. But mostly, thyroid hormones control the metabolic rates for your body at rest, the muscle tone that burns excess calories or the extra fat will deposit on your belly, your thighs, and your butt.

The **gut hormones** such as ghrelin, incretins (GLP-1 & GIP), cholecystokinin, glucagon, and other hormones produced in the stomach and intestine of the digestive system affect the appetite on a moment's notice and are strongly affected by food. Let's see how the hormones work in the cascade for fueling our metabolism.

DOCTOR TAI'S IMPORTANT TIP

Never walk around hungry! Hunger is a SOS signal from the brain, and it means that some chemical part of your body is ready for food. If you don't eat something, hopefully a nutritious snack, your body will think it is in starvation season. The body changes by conserving energy

& depositing fat. You will have big problems! It is far better to eat and drink something healthy to satisfy the longing when you sense the hunger pangs, rather than ignore it. How about an 8-ounce glass of ice tea (no sugar) and a salad until you are satisfied? Here are some great snacks to squelch the hunger voice: Nuts, raw vegetables, or a cup of chicken or vegetable broth or soup.

Important...always eat something in **reasonable quantity** and stop for ten minutes before eating again; stop for another 10 minutes and do it again until all hunger vanished. It **takes 20 to 30 minutes** for the stomach messengers to tell your brain you had enough and can stop now. BUT if you keep eating non-stop, the messages get to the brain TOO Late... you already ate too much! Give food a chance for the brain to register.

How Appetite Works

Keep in mind that the body's evolutionary job is to keep us from starving because the body needs a continuous, fresh supply of energy. **The purpose in eating, then, is to provide nutrition in the form of food to survive.** Food is digested and converted to energy, fuel for the body's cells.

Appetite science involves the communication between the brain and the gut and the regulation of metabolism. The brain and endocrine glands make hormones that oversee the appetite control system, regulate fat cells, control metabolism, and affect the digestive system.

Taste Preferences: We developed taste preferences as children when we liked sweetness or saltiness or other flavors, and the pleasure center of the brain was activated. This triggers the digestion process:

• The mesolimbic area in our brain center activates the stomach's digestion.
• The pancreas produces insulin.
• The liver processes the starches, fats and sugars we ate.
• This neural circuit set up a pathway for pleasure, and this is associated with eating what tasted good!

Hunger: What makes us hungry is a gut hormone called **ghrelin**. If you eat on a specific schedule, your body learns the schedule and ghrelin, the hunger hormone, anticipates and reminds us, like an alarm clock, that we feel the empty stomach and want to eat. Even the pancreas starts production of insulin in anticipation of food at the appointed hour.[14]

Next, the gut releases twin hormones called **incretins** in response to food. The twin hormones, **glucagon-like-peptide-1 (GLP1)** and **glucose dependent insulinotropic peptide (also known as GDIP)** tell the pancreas to ramp up insulin production.

Hunger centers exist in the hypothalamus as well as in other brain areas responsive to hormones like leptin, adiponectin, insulin, thyroid and others.

So when we feel hungry, ghrelin levels have increased and send the signal to the brain saying, "Eat." Ghrelin levels have decreased when we are no longer feeling hungry. Your hunger responds quickly to ghrelin levels.

• *In gastric bypass surgery, doctors cut out a part of the stomach to lower ghrelin. A smaller stomach and reduced ghrelin level help to decrease appetite.*

• *Higher levels of ghrelin promote eating. Secretion of growth hormone increases ghrelin levels and stimulates growth hormone.*

[14] Schwartz M.W. et al "Central nervous system control of food intake." Nature 404(2000): 661-72.

- *Your stomach secretes ghrelin every half hour, sending impulses to your brain. However, dieting stimulates production every twenty minutes.*

- *Ghrelin levels are higher when your body wants food. It's impossible to resist the biology of your body.*

- *When you finally give in and eat, your full stomach lowers ghrelin levels, reducing your appetite.*

- *When it comes to biology, you're going to lose that battle every time. NPY and CART fighting for the domination of your satiety center is the success or failure of your weight control war.*

Ghrelin

Satisfaction: Since we don't intend to eat ourselves into oblivion, three more hormones kick in to slow down eating. The nerves in the stomach and intestines register the "stretching" of our organ help to signal "full" caused by a peptide, **cholecystokinin (CKK)**, *that signals satiation in the brain.* However the signal lasts a brief time until the next meal. We may not register the "full" communication if your receptors are insensitive and resistant.

I'm Stuffed!

Next, the phenomenal regulating system sends two more hormones, **GLP-1** and **PYY**, to *the brain to say, "stop" and reduces the hunger feeling.* Here's the kicker, the stomach is not supposed to send more food further along because the body cannot digest it. **When the lower gut says, "Please quit," and we don't, then eating backfires on us.**

What the heck! Maybe it is a birthday or holiday like Thanksgiving and you stuff your face on this day. The stomach pushes the food along, but the body can't digest the food properly. Five hours later, you still feel like the turkey you stuffed.

*Here's another kicker: Because of the stuffed food, the **GLP-1** hormone adjusts your blood chemistry and the pancreas releases insulin, which absorbs the sugars of the foods and stores those excess sugars in the fat banks. Just one meal of being over stuffed, and the whole system of hormone communication is messed up! And you are on your way to a pound heavier and an inch wider at the waist or butt.*

We overeat because the appetite center of the brain, the hypothalamus, doesn't register the message that the stomach is full. However, the marvelous communication system for appetite has one more card up its sleeve. What happens when we get to the point of packing on the fat stores?

Suppression

In a normal functioning system, rather than allowing over-eating, fat itself produces a hormone called **leptin**, a longer acting hormone that circulates in the blood according the proportions of fat in the body. *Fat releases* **leptin** *into the bloodstream, and it travels to the hypothalamus, the same region that ghrelin targets, and signals appetite suppression if everything is functioning normally.*

☞ *More fat produces more leptin and less fat…less leptin. As an appetite suppressant, leptin regulates metabolism and energy intake.*

In other words, the satiation cue also revs up the nervous system and other body systems to metabolize food to fuel and give us energy.

DOCTOR TAI'S IMPORTANT TIP

Because leptin receptors respond to sweetness, leptin rewards sugar cravings, which the brain programs as a **learned addiction** *into your biochemistry.* [15] *Without the leptin red light to stop eating, our metabolism never gets the green light to convert food to fuel.*

Take L-carnitine 3 grams a day to help muscles to be more efficient in the use of carbohydrates.

Fructose blunts the satiety center because it tricks your mind so you stay hungry and continue to eat.

A small bowl of fiber fills you up and slows down the transit time of the gut.

I Can't Receive Your Signals – Receptor Resistance

> *Chronic excess eating raises the blood level of triglycerides, which can prevent leptin from reaching the brain.*

This is called **Leptin Receptor resistance. BIG PROBLEM!** *With the brain not receiving any fat and food signals of leptin, the body then thinks it is starving.[16] Overeating clogs the fat stores, signaling the liver to increase cholesterol.[17]*

> *You can see that the more we overeat, the hormones' receptors progressively become **less sensitive** or **insensitive**, and the chemicals in the body quit communicating with each other. The leptin receptors in the brain and other organs say to leptin, "Sorry, I don't get your message any more." And you continue to overeat and progressively making the condition worse.*

It is just like a teenager, who becomes accustomed to a screaming mother telling him to clean his room. He turns off to her message...signaling, "I don't get your message." Mom may scream louder and longer, but she becomes exhausted at the effort and gives up. Like leptin receptor cells, the kid never responds to the message. Like clogged receptor cells, the kid never cleans up his room. We could call this a "teenager resistance" or "teenager insensitivity." The same as applies to hormone **"leptin resistance"** or **"leptin insensitivity"**

In the next chapter, I wish to share more about the leptin hormone as a key player in this whole fat process, as well as leptin resistance and the connection to states of distress, inflammation and disease.

---

[15] Wang, GJ. "Similarity between obesity and drug addiction as assessed by neurofunctional imaging: a concept review." J of Addict. Disorders, (2004), 23(3): 39-53

[16] Banks, WA, et al. "Triglycerides induce leptin resistance at the blood-brain barrier." Diabetes. (2004) May, 53(5): 1253-60.

[17] Shmano, H. "Stenol regulatory element-binding protein family as a global regulator of lipid synthetic genes in energy metabolism." Vitam. Horm (2002); 65: 167-94

Chapter Ten

THE LEAP TO LEPTIN

The Leptin Discovery

In 1950, a research laboratory in Bar Harbor, Maine, had a strain of mice that were obese, lethargic, constantly hungry and insulin resistant. The fact that the mice were obese was unusual, but even more so that they exhibited the array of symptoms. This first report prompted further research into the obese mouse **blueprint**.

A gene called **ob** was discovered as responsible for the condition of the mice being diabetic, obese and living in a state of hunger. In the 1970s, scientist Doug Coleman discovered **the product of ob gene is the lack of** a hormone called **leptin** for the Greek work leptos meaning thin.[18] Next, when the mice were given leptin, they responded well in losing weight and regulating insulin. Leptin, as well as another protein called **adiponectin**, were the first of many fat cell hormones to be found.

> *However, leptin didn't turn out to be the panacea that everyone hoped, and more than 10,000 papers on leptin in thirteen years have explored this hormone's extensive relationship to other hormones and humans' overweight biochemistry.*

Leptin's Evolutionary Role

Leptin has been vital for human survival throughout the generations from prehistoric times. *This hormone prevented humans from dying of starvation when we were living in caves and hunting animals for a miserable, inconsistent living.* Until very recently, starvation had been the major cause of death for human beings.

In the grand timeline of human existence, it has been only a millisecond since food became as plentiful as it is now. Our body survival functions and hormones haven't had time

---

[18] Coleman, D.L. 1973. "Effects of Parabiosis of Obese with Diabetes and Normal Mice." Diabetologia 9:294-98.

to catch up. If our fat stores are low and we risk starvation, a body's leptin levels will be low, and all our metabolic survival tricks kick in to protect our body from dying by lowering metabolism and conserving (calories) energy to keep our body's weight up.

In this century of food abundance, there is a modern epidemic of obesity, when the body becomes overweight, leptin doesn't work right, nor does it protect us from obesity the way it protects us from starvation.

Also, this single leptin hormone communicates with a whole switchboard of other hormones. The role of leptin extends beyond appetite, metabolism, and body weight. **Leptin interacts with ALL other hormones like insulin, glucagon, growth hormone, thyroid hormone, testosterone, estrogen and cortisol.** It also plays a role in the growth of blood vessels and bones. Leptin further acts as a growth factor... as a regulator of puberty and fertility...as an immune system regulator.

So you can see that if we are overweight and obese with leptin abnormality and dysfunction of this very important hormone, it causes extensive problems in all aspects of our body physiology. We end up so sick and miserable.

Leptin's Interface...Digestion and Metabolism

Fat cells (adipocytes) produce the leptin, which circulates in the blood according to the proportions of fat in the body. The more fat, the more leptin. Less fat means less leptin.

In normal functioning systems, leptin maintains our bodies lean form in two ways. **First, as an appetite suppressant, *leptin* signals the brain's satiety center located in the hypothalamus** to say the body is satiated. If we maintain an even diet, which nourishes our energy, then our leptin levels will elevate in the blood to signal the hypothalamus, the body is good and we are satisfied and have no starvation.

Second, leptin increases our ability to use fat stores as a source of energy. When we have plenty of fat cells and keep the rate of metabolism functioning at a higher level through exercise, then we are full of energy.

Leptin is a master hormone orchestrating the proper functions of all the other metabolic and sexual endocrine hormones, which, in turn, insure a healthy, thriving, energetic, powerful lean human body.

When your body no longer suffers the metabolic craving and leptin resistance problems, you'll feel less hungry, less often, and be more easily satisfied with less food per sitting because your satiety center and receptor sensitivity is operating normally.

DOCTOR TAI'S IMPORTANT TIP

There are well-balanced individuals that need to eat only once or twice daily. They're not hungry and don't require additional food. Some experts say that's not good for you, as one must eat 3 times a day. Others say you must eat 5 or even 6 times a day to be healthy.

However, not all people fall into those categories. Why would people eat only eat 2 or 3 meals a day when the body is crying for 4 or 5 meals a day?

I think they need detoxing with **THE CRAVING FACTOR**. *When people feel hungry more often, they should adjust what they eat and portion size accordingly. Customize your eating habits to your metabolic needs. Your body AND your diet will work harmoniously, and you won't feel hunger as often.*

The real key is to clean your receptor sites and restore the normal function of your satiety center to communicate effectively with your food signals.

Leptin Resistance

Leslie, at age fifty-five felt good, exercised, and worked as a paralegal, sometimes fifty hours a week. As she sat, day after day, in the legal library or at her computer, her fluffy white fat cells produced more and more leptin. On her low calorie diet, Leslie doesn't comprehend why she continues to gain weight.

In the chapter on fat cells, I reported that **fat is the only tissue** *in the body* **that grows** *and expands throughout your life. The amount of leptin you have correlates to the* **amount of your fat** *and the size of the fat cells.*

Leptin first presented a **paradox to researchers!** How could a hormone, which promotes slender and lean, be elevated in overweight and obese people? What made sense was that overloads of leptin eventually caused a burnout and resistance in the **leptin receptors** of the brain and other target organs.

> *Leptin receptors become so bombarded with overload, excess leptin that they cease responding. This is called* **leptin resistance**...*the leptin red light for "stop eating" no longer works.*

We overeat because the appetite center in the brain, the hypothalamus, is slow to get or doesn't pick up the *stop-eating* signal. Wow, when the leptin red light stops working, and the leptin green light overloads the hormone communication switchboard, other parts of the system don't work as well either. Leptin is critical for functions such as
- Regulating blood circulation,
- Preventing blood clots,
- Making new bone,
- Regulating body temperature, metabolism and reproduction. For example, an excessively obese woman whose leptin receptor receives too few leptin signals will stop menses; exactly the same as an emaciated or too skinny athlete that has no body fat also stop menses. ***So the moral of the story...it is not only about hormone production, but also receptor hormone resistance not allowing the tissue to receive the critical signals, the net effect is the same.***

Leptin Deficiency
As I said earlier, the modern human body does not know how to handle ***excess***, thus we have leptin resistance from chronic and excessive increased leptin circulating in the blood. The brain's leptin receptors becoming less and less sensitive, resulting in receptors that always ignore the leptin levels no matter how high they are.

Leptin deficiency occurs when there are not enough fat cells to produce leptin. For example this can occur in person with Anorexia Nervosa who does not eat enough food or keep it down for proper assimilation. One also might see leptin deficiency in extreme athletes who are very lean with little fat percentages.

The body's natural response to hormone deficiency and resistance is to produce excess hormones that are ignored by the receptor cells. Leptin deficiency and leptin resistance both have the same result since the brain thinks the body is still starving and we are still in a food shortage survival mode.

In the early stages of leptin resistance, fat cells ramp up leptin production and can overcome the resistance. However, they can't keep up with the leptin demand without eating more and more. That is the origin of the endless cravings and eating binges that can't stop until the box of chocolate is empty or the tub of ice cream is gone.

Thus you see the problem. Leptin levels are high, yet the body experiences a "relative" leptin deficiency due to **Leptin Receptor Resistance.** *Such conditions create added inflammation, which "injure numerous peripheral tissues, including liver, pancreas, platelets, vasculature, and myocardium."* [19]

Leptin & The *Set Point*

Leptin causes a craving and addiction for food. So higher leptin causes increased eating as it seeks those dopamine highs which neuroscience found in the brain's *addiction* center. The vicious cycle continues as dopamine causes excess craving for foods, rewarding the pleasure center.[20]

[19] Martin, S. et al. "Leptin Resistance: A Possible Interface of Inflammation and Metabolism on Obesity Related Cardiovascular Disease. J Am Coll Cardiol, 2008; 52:1201-1210, doi:10.1016/j.jacc.2008.05.060

[20] (Krugel, U. et al. Eur. J. Pharma, 2003, Dec 15:482, 185-7)

Our body weight is normally regulated to stay within a range like our body temperature is maintained around 98.7 degrees. Set point is the brain's opinion of how much you should weigh. Set point is universal for all animals, including humans, and is affected by

- Satiety
- Hunger
- Cravings
- Metabolism
- Energy level

*Leptin activity in the hypothalamus gland establishes a **Set Point** for the body's weight. Set point means that your body's metabolism adjusts itself to maintain a body-to-fat ratio within a ten-pound range.*

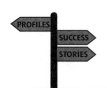
Karen's Story

For example, Karen was always comfortable at 115 pounds from the time she was in college all the way through her forties. Emergency surgery for the removal of an ovarian cyst left her in a state of nausea for ten days and her weight dropped to 90 pounds. As a result of the surgery, Karen developed inflammation patterns and sought homeopathic remedies from her health practitioner, who explained that her dehydrated cells and body might gain water and weight in balancing its health. Karen puffed up from a size two to a size twelve, and she was uncomfortable with the weight gain. Her body established a new set point of 140 pounds for Karen, and she couldn't lose her new set weight.

She felt her weight of comfort was 115, and strived to return to that point. Yet by the time she reached the higher weight, a new set point had been established, resisting all efforts to eat less and drop the undesired weight.

*Leptin receptors were set for the higher weight. What was she to do? Dieting only caused more discomfort, and the body went into the mode of conserving energy, leaving her still heavier than she desired and unable to drop the excess weight. She discovered that the **The Thin Factors**, Bauhinia, to clean and normalize sensitivity of the leptin receptors to improve metabolic burn, she used **Slimming Lyposome** transdermal cream for increased thermogenic burn of the fat cells. To improve craving, she used **Craving Factor**, a bound vitamin C with glutamine peptide, which readjusts the normal production of increasing CCK. It also lowers production of ghrelin by resurfacing the inner lining of the stomach and intestines. After only three months, she was able to lose 15 pounds, has more energy, and is on her way back to her desired weight and size.*

Chapter Eleven
How The Body Works

Lose weight! Feel great! Break the cycle!

"Dr Rich," as his patients called him, was a family practitioner on the east coast. He loved his work and patients and put in the long hours, sometimes not eating. Erratic eating habits and lack of exercise have added poundage to Dr. Rick's tall frame and expansive waistline. He had gastric bypass surgery, and still had food cravings. Before surgery, he thought his food cravings were caused by his bad psychology, poor eating habits, and long work hours.

After surgery, he understood that the intensive cravings were about hormonal imbalance. Dr. Rich sought a new route to deal with weight issues. He re-prioritized his intentions for health to include learning about the biochemistry of weight gain.

Dr. Rich's white adipose tissue (WAT) from his enlarged waist (omentum) and belly produced leptin, which also

- Regulates energy intake by creating hunger and sense of fullness in satiety.

- Cues energy output by increasing the metabolic rate or lowering the temperature of our body.

- This leptin capacity comes from collaboration with the thyroid function in creating the energy (ATP) within the mitochondria (battery) of the cells.

> *You have to stay in shape. My grandmother started walking five miles a day when she was 60. She's 97 today and we don't know where the hell she is.*
> *Ellen Degeneres*

Vicious Cycle of Excessive Eating

When the satiety center is not working normally with its usual sensitivity, the fullness hormone can't reach the hypothalamus. Why? Because excess eating raises the level of triglycerides (body gunk), which prevents leptin from reaching the brain, and the body thinks it is starving.[21]

Overeating clogs the fat stores, signaling the liver to increase cholesterol.[22]

You can see that the more we overeat, the greater the production of fullness (leptin) hormones in the blood, causing the satiety center hormone receptors to progressively become less sensitive. Like the screaming mother and her teenage son, the chemicals in the body quit communicating with each other. What a vicious cycle of excess and erratic eating that caused Dr. Rich to elect surgery, and then continue to feel the cravings and want to gorge on a heavy meal!

The doctor retrained his eating habits and tricked the craving by eating smaller low fat meals with protein or meals and lots of non-starchy vegetables to feel satisfied. That took great creativity in lifestyle remodeling.

---

[21] Banks, WA, et al. "Triglycerides induce leptin resistance at the blood-brain barrier." Diabetes. (2004) May, 53(5): 1253-60.

[22] Shmano, H. "Stenol regulatory element-binding protein family as a global regulator of lipid synthetic genes in energy metabolism." Vitam. Horm (2002); 65: 167-94

Rules of Thumb

Saturated fats you can eat in small amounts – virgin coconut oil and avocado. (Watch for high calories when eating too much)

Non-saturated fats, only olive oil is fit for human consumption. Better yet? Omega 3. Take 2 gel caps (enteric coated) 20 minutes before each meal for greater Satiety. Also full lignins from cold press virgin flax seed.

Enter the solution…**bauhinia**, which returns the *clean leptin receptors to their efficient signaling of the satiety center's hypothalamus* that we have had enough to eat.

Bauhinia's powerful antioxidants clean and rejuvenate the leptin receptor sites in the brain and open normal, efficient communication. With normal functioning receptor sensitivity, our switchboard for hormones is running smoother now. The lower levels of leptin volumes in the blood are ready to signal fullness to the satiety center, telling us to stop eating because we are happy with the amount of consumed calories. No fighting fat or willpower necessary!

Consider also using "**Craving Factor**" appropriately formulated of vitamin C bound to a glutamine peptide to normalize a higher level of CCK and longer ghrelin. Use transdermal **Slimming Lyposome** to increase thermogenic burn of fat cells around the stomach, upper thigh and butts.

Summary-How the Body Speaks

*In a **normal body**, when we eat, fat cells release leptin into the blood stream and leptin tells the brain, "I'm full. Quit eating. All energy levels are good."*

> *If we are **slightly overweight**, our leptin levels are too high and say, "Hey, body. Go burn some calories and extra fat, would you?"*

> *If we are **grossly overweight to obese**, leptin levels are so high that the leptin banging on our satiety center's receptor sites short-circuit. We don't get any warning at all. There is no red light or feeling over-stuffed. Our receptor sites in the brain are clogged, saying, "Hey green light, buddy. Pig out time!"*

Leptin's job is to save the human race from starvation. In the land of plenty, however, leptin's powerful influence on the adrenals' cortisol hormones, thyroid hormones and sex hormones can fuel compulsive, aggressive and addictive behaviors like sugar craving, midnight potato chips orgies and to-kill-for ravenous raids on the refrigerator.

Chronic stress can cause weight gain, even if you eat healthy and diet well. The reason is that persistent cortisol increases the circulation of blood sugar…glucose. The result is insulin overproduction to attempt to lower blood sugar, which diminishes the cells receptors sensitivity to insulin. The cells become insensitive to insulin, and therefore don't see that supply of glucose and excess insulin, which circulates in our blood stream. The continued elevation of circulating insulin and inefficient utilization of sugar leads to Type 2 diabetes.[23]

Cortisol and insulin play off of each other. In addition, chronic stress can lead to heart problems, diabetes, cancer, depression and other disease states. Even worse, evidence-based science show how stress is robbing your libido and lowering testosterone production, making you weaker and more like a functional *eunuch*.[24]

---

[23] Rizza, R. "Cortisol induced insulin resistance in man," J Clin Endo Met 54(1982):131

[24] Nielsson, P. et al. "Adverse effects of psychosocial stress on gonadal function and insulin levels in middle aged males", J Int Med 237 (1995):479)

Leptin Resistance and Insulin Resistance

Let me reiterate the pathway that produces obesity related illnesses and move to a discussion of inflammatory conditions:

- Our over-eating leads to abnormal (too high) leptin activity.

- It results in satiety center insensitivities called leptin resistance.

- So we stay hungry and store more fat rather than burning it (body thinks we are in starvation mode).

- High leptin means our fat stores too much sugar, and become engorged and plump, laden with triglycerides, which accumulate in the blood.

- Adipocytes, fat cells, do not absorb the free fatty acids and high sugars circulating in our blood, the result which causes insulin resistance to start in peripheral tissues like muscle. [25]

- We develop abnormal sugar metabolism from insulin receptor resistance leading to excess blood sugar. [26]

- When the increased sugar levels in blood become chronically high, we continue to store fat and have elevated sugar, insulin resistance, and later…high blood pressure, heart disease and accelerated aging, resulting in premature death. [27]

---

[25] Kraegen, EW & Cooney, GJ. Free Fatty Acids and Skeletal Muscle Insulin Resistance." Curr Opin Lipidol. (June, 2008) 19 (3), pp 235-241.

[26] (Reaven, G. et al."Non ketotic diabetes mellitus: insulin deficiency or insulin resistance?" Amer.J. Med. 60(1976):80.

[27] Brownlee, M. "Biochemistry and molecular cell biology of diabetic complications," Nature 414(2001):813.

Chapter Twelve

IT'S NOT ABOUT THE SUGAR

When you understand the mystery of physiology and the foundation of biology, you'll know what to do and why you're doing it...to rejuvenate your body. You can't fix something until you know what's wrong.

Insulin's Role

Remember when I said that our bodies don't handle the excesses of our modern world. In our ancestral history, leptin's job was to keep us from starving. Insulin also had a job...to keep sugar in our blood moving into active cells for energy. Good sources of sugar might have been seasonal fruits, and the person's work, movement and activity burned the blood sugar. Today, as then, the hormones cortisol, epinephrine, norepinephrine, glucagon, and growth hormone make sure that we always have some glucose available to the tissues that need it.

Insulin's role *then, as human history defined it, was not to lower blood sugar, but to convert food (sugar) to energy; and if there is extra, to direct it to storage.*

After each meal, the pancreas releases the insulin hormone to carry glucose to the body's cells. Insulin turns glucose (what we call sugar) from our food into energy. Like our cells need water and oxygen, they also need glucose for survival and energy production. Insulin resistance (IR) is the body's inability to respond to insulin's effects, for which the body compensates by creating more of the hormone.

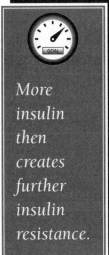

More insulin then creates further insulin resistance.

Notice that this vicious circular effect of insulin resistance is similar to that of leptin resistance. *When it is the perception of the cell receptors that they don't receive enough, they signal the brain that there is an equivalent hormone deficiency. The body gears up for more production even though the body has plenty of hormones, but it just isn't getting into the insensitive or resistant receptor.* Muscle cells lose their responsiveness to insulin and become resistant, like leptin-resistant brain cells lose their responsiveness to leptin.

> *Now that glucose molecules cannot enter the muscle cells and tissue, the sensitive liver converts sugar molecules to free fatty acids. (Fat cells enter the picture again!) Our blood dutifully carries the fatty acids right to the fat banks for storage. Whoops...fat stores respond with more leptin production, thus leptin resistance escalates.*

The snowball effect is now in a full-blown cycle...moving to next level of inflammatory phase conditions. When the body's production of insulin cannot keep up, hyperglycemia, too much sugar in the blood, will occur, and this most likely progresses to type 2 diabetes.

Fat Cells

Obese people and you have the same number of fat cells; the difference is the size of these fat cells. You don't become overweight

because you make more fat cells, but the fat globules swell each fat cell and increase your body size

When we hit the inflammatory state, the bodies are screaming, "Wake up, you! Your inner body conditions need to be balanced and cared for immediately because you are in the early stage of disease. There is still time to regroup, heal and get healthy…but if you don't…."

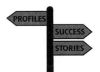 *Inflammation symptoms are like a middle stage between feeling fatigued and out of balance and moving to a disease state. We are already approaching disease by the time inflammation symptoms flare up.*

A thorough discussion of inflammation is in the next chapter, but Christopher's story shows you how one life event can cause health to shatter overnight.

PROFILES
SUCCESS
STORIES

Christopher's Story

*Few of us realize that we have insulin resistance (**IR**). Symptoms don't just pop up and say hello. **IR** can be years in the making as was the case with Christopher when a stressful life event triggered his full-blown diabetes.*

He completed two tours of Vietnam as a young man, returned home to marry, entered his father's printing business and settled down. Years passed with six children, thirteen grandchildren and a sedentary, happy life. His exercise was golf on Sundays, and over thirty years, the lean Marine's body gained weight around the middle, despite the fact that he thought of himself as an active, healthy person. He may have been active, but he wasn't fit!

The most stressful event of his life, "even more than the war," in his words, was when the new owner of his father's legacy ran the printing business into the ground. The profits shares owed to Christopher ceased to exist. Within three weeks, Christopher developed diabetes, and he felt, "110 years old."

His waist-circumference measurement indicated leptin resistance, probably twenty years in the making. He may have noticed being light-headed or tired on the golf course, and chalked it up to stress and aging. Meantime, he enjoyed his strawberry ice cream several times a week as well as morning coffee and his wife's home cooked meals. In other words, his food intake was routine for his adult life. For a family of the 60s and 70s, Christopher and his wife thought they were eating well and enjoyed a convenient lifestyle. They wouldn't have noticed the changing ingredients in processed foods to high fructose corn syrup, trans fats and excitotoxins.

Unlike Christopher, we can no longer afford to be uninformed! To thrive, generations today must learn about exercise, eat nutritious foods and definitely take the supplements that support great health!

When he was diagnosed, Christopher called a family meeting to inform nineteen other people (children and grandchildren) that they might be at risk. Doctors call *type 2 diabetes a lifestyle disease, and they also believe a genetic component is at play. What we do for our health today means that we model and do for the next generations.*

Here is how it worked out in his six children's lives. One of Christopher's children had hypoglycemia (which is often the first stage before Hyperglycemia). Both sons grew huge waistlines in their early fifties; golf being their exercise weekly, just like their Dad. Two of his daughters married men with diabetes, significantly increasing their children's chances for diabetes. Three of Christopher's granddaughters had gestational diabetes, gained significant weight at pregnancy, and haven't lost it. One has already developed diabetes in her early forties, and the other two, who are in their mid-thirties, took the hint and started exercise and weight loss programs.

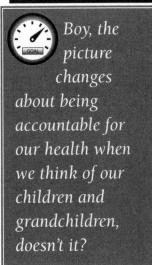

Boy, the picture changes about being accountable for our health when we think of our children and grandchildren, doesn't it?

Being at risk for health issues starts years before we see the actual disease itself. People who are overweight to obese have high levels of both insulin and leptin. Their bodies try to overcome the resistances with higher production of more hormone and they might notice mild symptoms.

Improving receptor functions and alleviating the resistance happens through a

combination of exercise,
proper diet, metabolic
balance, liver and bowel
cleansing and brain
satiety rejuvenation with
bauhinia...all of which
you'll find in the section
four **guides** *to your health.*

Risk Factors

Leptin resistance from fat cells and insulin resistance always occur together. The more risk factors you have, the more severe the insulin resistance can be. Fat cells become less responsive to insulin. [28] The risk factors below include physical issues as well as contributing lifestyle factors. I believe the last factor of stress is probably way overlooked by the general public.

Christopher, for instance, couldn't have predicted the business failure or influenced another man's decision. However, he could have had stress management techniques, even as simple as deep breathing or walking a dog, that helped him adapt or cope better. What are your routines for managing stressors? Read the exercise section very carefully if you see yourself reflected in the list below. These risk factors are

[28] Hirosumi,J. et al. "A central role for JNK in obesity and insulin resistance", Nature 420(2001):333.

indicative of leptin resistance, insulin resistance **and** type-2 diabetes.

- Chronic pain
- Fat in the belly (visceral fat)
- Genetics
- Infection or illness
- Inflammation
- Kidney problems
- Leptin resistance
- Liver problems
- Low potassium levels
- Menopause
- Mental illness
- Obesity or being overweight
- Physical inactivity
- Poor diet
- Pregnancy
- Puberty
- Smoking
- Stress

DOCTOR TAI'S IMPORTANT TIP

The best way to determine your risks for insulin resistance, aka Metabolic Syndrome, is to measure your waist. The broader your waist circumference, the more layers of inner fat have developed within you. Men whose waists are over 40 inches and women who measure larger than 36 inches have one highly significant risk factor. If you are not physically active, start moving your body! Simply walking at a brisk pace three to five times each week for at least 20 minutes will help.

Smart supplementations, like bauhinia, chromium, Cordyceps full spectrum and DHEA will also help.

(See www.healthsecretsUSA.com)

Just like leptin resistance and insulin resistance go hand in hand, so have doctors been aware that diabetes and cardiovascular problems occur in tandem. Research studies have linked the disturbances in insulin resistance with other cardiovascular symptoms.

Insulin regulates cellular nourishment, and to have resistance to insulin sends our metabolisms into a downward spiral. Metabolic diabetes means having insulin receptor insensitivity to regulate cell energy nutrition. Also contributing to the situation are lack of physical activity and visceral fat, poor diet, hormonal loss from andropause or menopause, or some physical (illness) and emotional shock (business) like Christopher experienced.

> Now that the link between leptin resistance and insulin resistance is clear, we've clustered risk factors together and called it the **Metabolic X Syndrome**. Other symptoms around obesity, such as high blood pressure, high lipid levels and high blood sugar, **affect 22% of the American population.**

Obesity elevates blood pressure because of the negative effect on lipid levels, higher cholesterol and high triglycerides, all of which trigger **inflammation**.

You have Metabolic Syndrome if you have at least three risk factors.[29] *Risk factors for Metabolic Syndrome **are not the causes of disease**, but are associated as a typical cluster of symptoms. Having more risk factors increases the severity of the condition.*

---

[29] Bruni, A. et al. "Does leptin play a cytokine-like role within the airways of COPD patients?" European Respiratory Journal. September, 2005: 32, 1231-1236.

So think of risk factors as warning signs. These factors are what your doctor will be looking for, so you should know them also. Some doctors label insulin resistance and metabolic syndrome as the same thing.

As you read these factors you'll recognize that they are all symptoms of every subject we've discussed thus far: *overeating, being inactive, being overweight or obese, having visceral fat stores, developing leptin resistance and then insulin resistance...* all part of our behaviors which signal your hormonal switchboard is clogged with mixed signals.

- Fat or weight around the middle. Men, measure your waistlines, and if you register greater than 40 inches, consider the health plan in section four. Same for you ladies if your waist measurement is greater than 35 inches.

- High blood pressure (138/85 mm Hg or higher)

- High blood sugar (fasting blood sugar of 110 mg/dL or greater)

- High fat in blood (triglyceride)

- Low good cholesterol (HDL level less than 50 mg)

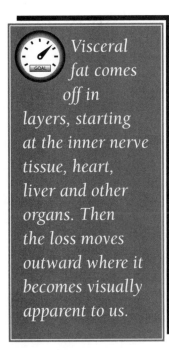

Visceral fat comes off in layers, starting at the inner nerve tissue, heart, liver and other organs. Then the loss moves outward where it becomes visually apparent to us.

These risks increase with age and gained body fat. As obesity increases in the United States, more than half of the adult population and a growing number of children are at risk for grave health issues.

Metabolic Syndrome and Fat

Visceral adiposity refers to the fat cells around the (omentum) internal organs. Visceral = inner, adiposity = fat.

This white fat (WAT) is responsible for patterns of hormone resistance. WAT cells in your belly increase cortisol, the stress hormone, and decrease growth hormone. This decrease lowers testosterone in men and estrogen in women, and causes flabby muscles without tone. You feel weak and have muscle cramps. Visceral fat cells produce even more toxic hormones, spewing inflammation and resulting in leptin and insulin resistance that hinder your health.

Type 2 Diabetes

Twenty-five per cent of the people with insulin resistance go on to develop full-blown diabetes, known as type-2 diabetes.

When someone with insulin resistance eats a meal that is high in sugar or processed carbohydrates, the pancreas pumps out too much insulin. This causes a sudden and rapid blood sugar fall, causing symptoms like rapid heartbeat, shakiness, dizziness, sweating, or blurred vision.

More than 80% of people with type 2 diabetes are overweight. Type 2 diabetes is a condition where the body produces enough insulin, but the individual suffers insulin receptor resistance.

Insulin resistance makes fat cells produce more TNF-cx, a toxic hormone that causes inflammation. Excess fat, especially in the belly, causes insulin resistance, leptin resistance and elevated blood sugar, leading to thyroid resistance and high blood pressure, as well as increased blood clotting and increased inflammation throughout the body.

Insulin resistance means that the receptors at the surface of the cell are blind to the presence or effects of insulin. The fat cell responds by producing excess free fatty acids, which cause a condition called lipotoxicity that worsens insulin resistance.

Elevated insulin stimulates the production of excess fat in the abdomen, in muscles, and inside organs. These hormones cause both leptin resistance, cortisol excess resistance and insulin resistance, resulting in thyroid resistance. ***The cycle perpetuates weight gain, low energy and low metabolism.***

Round & Round We Go

In summary, many people who are overweight have elevated cortisol levels, which make you gain weight. ***The cycle continues with excess fat in the belly producing hormonal imbalance, leptin resistance, leading to thyroid resistance, insulin resistance and cortisol excess.*** Toxic fat cell hormones stimulate the adrenal gland to pump out more cortisol.

Now you can see that the process of hormones sending signals to receptors on cells is delicate. If one hormone like leptin becomes deficient, then its ability to communicate with the satiety center in the brain's hypothalamus and the large number of other metabolic hormones goes awry.

(See protocol: Stage I diet)

Chapter Thirteen

INFLAMMATION

What Is Inflammation?

The last several chapters have opened our eyes to the inflammatory shock that coexists with hormonal communication confusion. The hormonal cascades involved in the delicate processing of food into energy have opportunities for miscues, causing metabolic disorders. While we have focused on leptin resistance and insulin resistance, another powerful damaging process called inflammation is going on in our bodies as our immune system works overtime to strengthen inner resources.

Inflammation is the first response of the immune system to infection, irritation or trauma.

Inflammation that once helped us survive bites, stings, and accidents, can go awry in the modern world. When inflammation, the body trying to correct an imbalance, fires too long and hard, then a chronic inflammation causes its own problems like attacking organs, muscles, and joints.

Doctors label inflammation with an "itis" word according to the organs, tissues, vessels or other parts that are involved. Here are a few examples:
- Liver inflammation = hepatitis
- Colon inflammation = colitis
- Joint inflammation = arthritis
- Heart inflammation – myocarditis
- Sinus inflammation - sinusitis
- Stomach inflammation – gastritis

Have you noticed how one person with arthritis has good days and bad days with pain? Or how someone with a low-grade fever feels as if the flu clutches their abdomen one afternoon, and then they are up and moving the next morning?

One inflammation trait is that the pain increases or decreases depending upon the level of tissue insult or toxicity, the balance of the body's systems.

DOCTOR TAI'S IMPORTANT TIP

Inflammation Markers

There are several tests you can take to determine the level of inflammation in your body. An extra protein, **C-reactive protein**, is released from the site of an injury. The protein then circulates in the bloodstream and is measured as a marker of inflammation, usually associated with heart disease.

A **C-reactive protein (CRP) blood test** can be performed along with a cholesterol test.

Ask for an hs.CRP level.

Under 1.0 milligrams per liter of blood means you have a low risk; 1.0 to 2.9 milligrams indicates your risk is intermediate

More than 3.0 milligrams is high risk.

Another test is a **fasting blood insulin level.** This test is used to screen for diabetes and heart disease, and used also a marker for inflammation. The higher your insulin levels are, the more inflammation your body is likely to produce.

Like the cluster of symptoms for Metabolic X syndrome, inflammation exists in conjunction with being overweight or obese, having cardiovascular problems, diabetes, smoking, long-term infections and stress. Are you starting to see the bigger picture here about hormone communication and their maintenance of youthful metabolism?

We have to become like vigilant soldiers on night watch, observing what we eat, how the body feels, and being disciplined in our exercise routines to offset inflammation.

The next section explores more of the research on the relationship of inflammation to other Metabolic X symptoms to demonstrate the inter-relationships of hormones communications or lack thereof.

Chronic Inflammation Affects Hormones

In his book, *The Fat Resistance Diet*, Leo Galland, MD. explains that chronic inflammation throws hormones that protect your health into disarray. Two immune system molecules, which reduce inflammation, also interfere with cells' receptors receiving leptin's signals.

👉 *"Two specific molecules, SOCS-1 and SOCS-3, are called suppressors of cytokine signaling (SOCS). In animal studies, the molecules jam the signals that leptin is supposed to deliver to brain cells and muscle cells."* [30]

Inflammation's Role in Leptin Resistance

Leptin hormone, produced by adipose tissue, is involved in several diseases, one being chronic obstructive pulmonary disease (COPD). Researcher, Andreina Bruno and colleagues studied the correlation between leptin, its receptor, and inflammation in three populations: smokers with COPD, smokers without COPD and non-smoking healthy volunteers. The authors found a direct correlation between leptin's presence in bronchial tissue and the progressive functional impairment in COPD. They considered leptin's presence an inflammation marker,[31] leading one to feel severe fatigue, lack stamina, and have chronic painful muscles and bouts of depression.

Inflammation, Obesity and Heart Problems

In another study, heart specialists found the link of obesity to chronic heart inflammation. They tested and tracked the development of heart failure in 7000 men and women of diverse ethnicities.

They found that obese persons had higher blood levels of interleukin 6, C-reactive protein and fibrinogen, which are all immune system proteins involved in inflammation.

---

[30] Galland, L. MD, The Fat Resistance Diet, Unlock the Secret of the Hormone Leptin to: Eliminate Cravings, Supercharge Your Metabolism, Fight Inflammation, Lose Weight & Reprogram Your Body to Stay Thin. New York: Broadway (December, 2006)

[31] Bruni, A. et al. "Does leptin play a cytokine-like role within the airways of COPD patients?" European Respiratory Journal. September, 2005: 32, 1231-1236.

> *"A near doubling of average interleukin 6 levels alone* **accounted for an 84 percent greater risk of developing** **heart failure in the study population.** *Similarly, a near tripling of average levels of C-reactive protein in obese study participants increased the chance of heart failure by 36 percent."* [32]

In 2005, researchers at the University of Buffalo showed the first solid evidence that mononuclear cells, a type of white blood cell that produces inflammation, are more likely to occur in obese patients at risk of developing heart disease and/or diabetes. The cells interfere with insulin production and create a precursor to atherosclerosis of the worse and often fatal kind called Unstable (bursting) Atheromas.

 Other researchers from the Methodist DeBakey Heart Center identified a molecular link between obesity and inflammation.

Their research demonstrated that a **high fat diet** leads cells to produce chemokines, molecules, which attract inflammatory white blood cells in fat tissue. This inflammation prevents the fat banks from storage and the fat floats in the bloodstream and goes to the muscles or liver, and starts the insulin and leptin resistance processes again.[33] The result is devastating diseases like Non-Alcoholic Fatty Liver becoming epidemic, leading to Liver Fibrosis and Liver Cirrhosis, which is nearly always fatal.

[32] Original Study) Kiang, Lie. PhD. Et al. Multiethnic study of atherosclerosis (MESA), sponsored by the National Heart, Lung, and Blood Institute. J Am Coll Cardiol, 2006; 48:2285-2292.

[33] Article URL: http://www.medicalnewstoday.com/articles/56997.php

Too many calories promote inflammation, and obesity feeds back to the neurons to further promote inflammation, even in our brain centers.

The brain's hypothalamus, which regulates appetite and energy balance, can be thrown off by an overload of calories by yet another molecule called IKKB/NF-B.[34] An out-of-whack hypothalamus starts the inflammatory chain reaction, resulting in leptin resistance and insulin resistance, resulting in thyroid resistance.

Going On and On

You have been patient as I've offered supportive research that links all the topics we have discussed thus far in *The Thin Factors*.

Obesity...inflammation...miscues in hormonal cell signals and receptors...leptin resistance...insulin resistance...thyroid resistance...Metabolic X...diabetes... cardiovascular disease... inflammation, brain allergies...

---

[34] Zhang, X. et al. "Hypothalamic IKK/NF-B and ER Stress Link Overnutrition to Energy Imbalance and Obesity." Cell Journal, (10-3-2008) Vol 135:1. Pp. 61-73

Aging adults as well as children aren't suffering from single diseases anymore, but have two, three or four conditions simultaneously.

Based on government survey data, 44 percent of Americans in 2005 had at least one chronic medical condition, which could include diabetes, high blood pressure, high cholesterol levels, cancer, arthritis, heart failure and others.

Does it not sound to you like the modern human body is on overload, and we've found leptin to play major roles in all of these conditions? Maybe the real illness is just called **Excesses of Modern Life?**

Many researchers link hormone miscues in cell signaling to *inflammation, leptin resistance, cortisol excess resistance and insulin resistance, resulting in thyroid resistance.* Having poor diets and being overweight precedes all. However, the conditions around food and exercise loom ever greater in importance when someone is only ten pounds overweight. Yet they may be in the 45th percentage for fat, and actually have the same problems as someone who is 50 or 100 pounds overweight.

Action needs to be taken because the whole health issue hinges on hormones' abilities to communicate. *The Thin Factors* (*Bauhinia*) is a tremendous help in cleaning cell receptors as promoting the loss of inches of abdominal fat. (See protocol: Stage I)

There are answers!

Cleansing the resistant receptor cells (Insulin, Leptin, and Thyroid) to work normally again, and boosting thyroid, leptin, adiponectin and other fat cell hormones, improves every aspect of our lives. Our bodies become leaner and more efficient.

Excessive hunger and cravings diminish, and metabolism works toward the body achieving a healthy weight. With the resulting increase in energy, we experience better moods, more restful sleep and have a clearer mind. Hormonal balance, then, simply translates to feeling better, stronger and living longer.

Our cells absolutely must speak to each other and be clearly understood. When a hormone or protein knocks on a cell's door, the receptor must be able to open the door and let the chemical enter the cell in open communication. Without this process, we have no metabolism, energy or fuel for living. Cells die off one by one, and the system sends garbled signals to the brain, leading to severe craving and suffering from Satiety Center resistance.

While this may all seem so complicated, the solutions are so simple. The solutions start by taking **The Thin Factors** bauhinia before each meal, wash your digestive system with **Craving Factor,** start your lifestyle habits of basic exercise and implement and stick to a simple nutritious food eating plan. **Find your TOTAL solutions in Section V!**

Part IV

PARTNERSHIP BAUHINIA, SCIENCE & YOU

Chapter Fourteen

FROM THE AMAZON TO THE LAB

More Than Folk Medicine

Like me, other scientists and doctors have developed interests in the ancient folk medicines from Amazonia for the solutions they could offer modern societies. As I tramped through the mystical rain forest, my eye would not have noticed the legume bush with leaves like elephant ears called Bauhinia. The ancient medicine men must show us the way to rely on botanicals. Their knowledge has been passed from generation to generation for centuries.

> *The shaman stood next to the bush, which extended its branches to his shoulders. He tenderly touched the leaves, lifting them, placing his hand on it, comparing sizes. He continued his short lecture, "This tree that makes people well, is for skin sores and infections, diarrhea, a tonic for aging...*

The leaves of Bauhinia are boiled in teas and broths, which natives drink as a tonic for digestion and to soothe upset stomachs. Elders drink the broth as a stimulant. The plant is a diuretic with ingredients that fight fungus, bacteria and Candida. The natives prepare the bark as an antidote to diarrhea. The natives use Bauhinia extracts for snakebite treatments.

The Healing Tree also fights diabetes. One teaspoon of ground Bauhinia as a tea taken after eating helps to regulate blood sugar. Knowing this, my burning question was, "How could this plant also help with weight loss?"

Bauhinia Offers Relief

 Bauhinia cleans the cell receptors, which receive leptin and or insulin signals. Bauhinia heals leptin resistance and insulin resistance and reverses it. It can

also open the brain barrier to normalize satiation to stop cravings and excessive eating.

Bauhinia supplements or teas lower triglycerides as it affects the brain barrier, lowering inflammation and normalizing the natural body's response to leptin. You will functionally be more effective in stopping the addiction to overeating.

This whole process involving Bauhinia's influences allows our normal metabolism **to eat less, to burn fat and stop inflammation**. If you are an overeater or an unconscious eater, your eating can go awry with a series of small steps into overweight and obesity.

• *If you feel satiated, but choose one more, small helping, remember that the stomach and intestine's muscles become distended.*

• *Then, the food stops midway down and ferments because the molecules for digestion got overloaded.*

• *The stuck foods alert the pancreas to release insulin, and we end up with too much blood glucose.*

• *Perhaps you never feel satiated? So you continue to eat, causing fat stores to release more and more leptin until leptin resistance settles in.*

• *Or, you might eat well and don't exercise much. The lack of movement is just as disastrous to your health and overeating or not eating right.*

Do you see how many small choices we make throughout the process of health? Take a food inventory and determine what you eat or how you eat that triggers hormones that produce inflammation, which means our bodies enter a phase of disease, but we can still turn back the tide.

I learned much from the Native Elder about Bauhinia, and when I returned to the United States after my Ecuadorian adventures, I continued to learn.

Human Weight Loss Research

Previous studies have researched the medicinal effects on Bauhinia for antioxidant, analgesic, hypoglycemic, astringent, diuretic, blood cleanser, uterine relaxant, anti-aging toner, purgative, and anti-inflammatory properties. One small study by Pinto & Pinto[35] followed the weight variation in ten people who ingested 30 grams daily of Bauhinia extract in alcohol. Their lifestyle routines remained consistent. At the conclusion of the study, everyone had weight loss over the course of fifteen days, as shown below.

Gender	Age	Net Weight Loss
M	53	8.5 lbs
M	51	6 lbs
M	46	2 lbs
F	62	5 lbs.
F	54	3 lbs.
F	54	18 lbs.
F	53	14 lbs.
F	48	6 lbs.
F	32	4 lbs.
F	27	7 lbs.

Anti-Inflammatory Research

You've read in previous chapters that one significant result of being overweight or obese is inflammation.

 By the time a person recognizes and is diagnosed with inflammatory conditions, they are already on their way to a disease state.

35 Pinto F. & Pinto, M. I. "Bauhinia Tarapotensis as a Weight Loss Stimulant." Clinica De Especialidades Biorregenerativas, Ecuador. © 2008 Fundacion Omniversidad de Amerika, Ecuador.

Lucky for us the various types of Bauhinia have been tested and verified as healing for inflammatory conditions.

DOCTOR TAI'S IMPORTANT TIP

Uses for Bauhinia

Bauhinia's leaves have been used for conditions of inflammation and for decongestion (Cordero, 1950).[36]

If you have experienced sore throats or have difficulty in feeling bloated after a meal, a cup of Bauhinia tea before each meal soothes the inflammation.

The healing tree's bark is employed as an anti-diarrhea formula (Kohn, 1992).[37] *A cup of Bauhinia tea also works for this condition and cramping.*

A methanol extract of Bauhinia's leaves demonstrated antioxidant and radical scavenger properties (Braca, et.al. 2001).[38] *Our body is as clean as our blood, basically. The anti-oxidant properties of the Bauhinia capsules or teas help neutralize the blood's acidic properties.*

Research (Conner & Grisham, 1996)[39] *indicated free radicals produced by phagocytic leukocytes during inflammatory conditions and tissue injuries result in further inflammation and damage to our body.*

[36] Cordero, J. "Enumeracion de Botanica de los principales Plantas asi utiles come Nocivas, Indigenas o Aclimatadas, que se en la Provincias del Azuay y del Cahar de la Repibblica de Ecuador; Segunda Edicion Edit, Afrodisio Aguado, SA, Madrid, p. 251. (1950).

[37] Kohn E). La Cultura Medica de los Runas de laRegion Amazzonica Ecuadoriana; Hombre y Ambiente 21, Ediciones Abya-Yala, Ecuador. P. 105 (1992).

[38] Braca, A. et. al. "Antioxidant Principles from Bauhinia tarapotensis." J. Nat Prod 64:892-893. (2001)

[39] Conner, EM & Grisham, MB. "Inflammation, free radicals an antioxidants." Nutrition 12: 274-277. (1996).

The properties of the Bauhinia leaves for treatment of inflammatory conditions include triterpenic acids belonging to the ursane and oleababe series. Since you now know that inflammation is a precursor to serious disease states, imagine reducing inflammatory conditions and at the same time stopping appetite cravings with bauhinia!

Reduced Diabetic Symptoms

In addition to weight reduction and anti-inflammatory uses, Bauhinia has been the subject of studies in recent years using the plant's extracts in diabetes management.

In South American countries like Brazil and Ecuador, a tea from the Bauhinia leaves is used for diabetic treatment, usually by drinking a cup of tea after the meal.

Bauhinia candicans increases peripheral metabolism of glucose, which can be helpful in monitoring diabetes or hypoglycemic activity.[40] This type of knowledge helps us by giving us a choice to use pharmaceutical drugs or more natural options for managing disease states. I vote natural any day, rather than experiencing the side effects of drugs.

[40] Fuentes, O. et.al. "Hypoglycemic activity of Bauhinia candicans in diabetic induced rabbits. Fitoterapia. 75: pp 527-532, (2004).

The Thin Factors Solution

For all of the issues that start with being overweight, Bauhinia is an **evidence-based solution** that excites many of us doctors who seek the natural answers from Earth's botanicals. The results of several pilot studies yielded promising results!

Pilot Study: The results of a four-week pilot project, double blind study, which used bauhinia for weight loss in overweight people, was effective in its objective.[41] Eighteen men and thirteen women, assigned to either a treatment or a placebo group, took a "treatment" thirty minutes before each meal. The treatment group took a bauhinia leaf extract. Both groups received a vitamin/mineral supplement. The subjects were asked specifically not to intentionally change their diet or choice of food and/or exercise regiment, reason being that we wanted to see if they were capable of losing weight if the subjects did nothing but follow our Thin Factors supplement. Measurements of weight and circumference of hips, waist, and chest took place before and after the four-week study.

30-DAYS TRIAL RESULTS			
Group B – Treatment Group	**Initial Statistics**	**Final Statistics**	**Change**
Number – 14 **Males – 7** **Females - 7**	**Mean Age in Years = 54.3**		
Mean Weight	216.360	211.696	-4.661
BMI	32.350	31.793	-0.557
Waist (inches)	42.286	40.693	-1.593
Hips (inches)	46.214	44.893	-1.324
Waist to Hip Ratio	0.914	0.905	-0.008

A comparison of changes between the placebo group (a) and the treatment group (b) two revealed a statistically significant difference in the body mass index, which is

---

[41] Steelman, Morganstern, & Tai. "Bauhinia: A New Herbal substance for Weight Loss?" The Bariatrician (Summer 2008) pp.18-19.

interesting since the regular regimens for diet and exercise for each participant remained the same throughout the four weeks. Several subjects reported increased energy and a sense of well-being.

DOCTOR TAI'S IMPORTANT TIP

You could also replicate this study in your home.

Take your own weight and measurements of neck, upper arms, butt, upper thighs, hips, waist and chest.

Take a bauhinia capsule thirty minutes before you eat any meal. For those of you who are very overweight or a difficult case, **take two capsules 30 minutes before each meal.**

Do this every day for one month and then take retake your weight and circumference measurements.

Most likely you will notice some weight loss, but also the measurements will show your loss of fatty tissue.

Remember that we lose visceral fat first from the inside organs, so expect the inches to drop away.

Using our diet secrets and advice as well as exercise routine greatly enhances the weight loss and shrink inches away.

Improvement, like in the above study can be had at home by adding **Max Slim** *to increase metabolic resting burn rate,* **Slimming Lyposome** *cream to apply for spot fat burning thermogenic melt away when applied on stomach and thigh areas, and* **Craving Factor** *to rejuvenate the gut and intestinal inner lining and kick up hormone production to stop craving.*

Following Up! More Research...

After the successful first study, we continued to follow the subjects. Three men and five women from the treatment group continued taking Bauhinia in a non-double blind fashion. The report of this study published in *The Bariatrician*[42] indicated the participants took 5 milliliters or 200 mg of the extract prior to each meal. Once again, participants did not intentionally change their normal eating habits or any additional exercise. The mean weight of the group was 216.75 at week zero and 204.68 at week 8. The average net loss was 12.07 pounds per subject. The loss was also reflected in their circumference measurements:

- **Average waist circumference loss: 41.625 to 38.125 = Net loss = 3.5 inches**
- **Average hip circumference loss: 45.625 to 43.8125 = Net = 1.8125 inches**

The waist to hip ratio was reduced by .38 of an inch.

What phenomenal progress!

The Wonder of Bauhinia

Our lab HPLC has developed a proprietary bauhinia formulation and the patent is pending. Once the research showed us how bauhinia goes to work detoxifying the body and also cleansing and scrubbing cell receptors to better receive leptin hormone, we wanted to explain to you in this book. Why?

*Because the science of appetite is so new, really only a dozen years old, and we need to take fast action immediately before the **Globesity** epidemic overtakes us all.*

---

[42] Morganstern, S. MD. et. al. "Follow-Up Report: Continuing Significant Changes in Weight and Anthropometric Measurements with Open-Label Extension of Trial with Bauhinia Forficata. The Bariatrician (Fall, 2008) pp. 12-14.

Bauhinia's action on the metabolic system normalizes
physiological activity in these ways:

- **Normalizes the leptin hormone through neuropeptide Y (NPY). When this powerful appetite hormone Y rises, due to leptin resistance, a person eats uncontrollably.**

- **Regulates insulin resistance, which helps to normalize that inevitable roller coaster of very high and lows of blood sugar effects, and**

- **Adjusts adrenal hyperactivity by lowering adrenalin stimulation and cortisol overproduction from stress activities.**

- **Hundreds of polyphenols act positively on the heart and vascular system through cleansing of the liver. This lowers bad lipids/cholesterol, triglycerides, and harmful lipoproteins.**

- **Powerful antioxidants neutralize free radical attacks and slow down aging deterioration. There is even some evidence of reversal of aging. For example, white and gray hair spontaneously reverted to its original natural color.**

- **Neutralizing AGE, advanced glycation end product, a toxic crosslinking of glucose to protein that damages tissues and DNA, causing severe aging problems and lipofucsin discoloration of the skin and organs, which hallmarks old age.**

- **Cleans and lowers the blood brain barrier for normal hormonal activity on the satiety center, controlling the eating reflex, and stops craving for carbohydrates.**

Remember that the hormone ghrelin, along with incretins (GLP-1 & GIP), cholecystokinin, glucagon, and other hormones produced by the digestive system, affect the appetite on a moment's notice and are strongly affected by food. Ghrelin stimulates the appetite, and when it runs amuck, our food cravings, addictions really, seem never-ending.

*The Thin Factors, Bauhinia, and **Craving Factor** normalize production of those hormones to keep appetites aligned with the body's proper biochemistry. They normalize the high production of gut satiety hormones such as cholecystokinin (CCK), one of the most powerful anti-hunger hormones in the human body, giving that wonderful full sensation of satisfaction. **(See Total Protocol Stage I & Stage II)***

Without Bauhinia and **Craving Factor**, the peptide YY (PYY), that tells us that the stomach is full and distended, would not signal the satiety center properly. Without **The Thin Factors** and **Craving Factor**, it seems like we would just keep eating...and eating...and eating, developing that Buffet Syndrome.

So it takes a few days for **The Thin Factors** Bauhinia to repair these abnormal chronic problems. Patience in the first week pays off big dividends later.

*Also I have personally noticed that when I take double dose for a week or so at the beginning of my program, bauhinia and **Craving Factor** work in supporting these multiple digestive abnormalities to repair themselves.*

*Some people like to take Bauhinia 15 minutes before each meal, and others like it with their meal. Always take Bauhinia with ounces of water because Bauhinia must use the **Craving Factor** dissolved in 16 oz of water (4 times daily) or ice tea to be transported to the digestive tract and into the blood stream to work.*

Consistently, Bauhinia has been shown effective in weight loss and in helping the brain and body control appetite, clean leptin receptors, balance glucose and insulin, and reduce inflammation. When all is said and done, Nature could not have provided a more suitable, affordable solution for humans' modern-day issues with excess.

Imagine how the future of our children changes from bleak to bright as **The Thin Factors, Craving Factor,** and **Slimming Lyposome** cream offers an answer to overweight trends, obesity and its related health conditions and longer life trends! **(*Solutions in Section V*)**

Chapter Fifteen

Loving THE Healthy Lifestyle!

What I do today is important because
I am exchanging a day of my life for it.
Author Unknown

Get A Lifestyle

When psychologist Alfred Adler spoke of a person's style of life, he wouldn't foresee the variations of "lifestyles" we have today. Adler said, "The style of life of a tree is the individuality of the tree expressing and molding itself against the environment. We recognize a style when we see it against a background of an environment different from what we expect, for then we realize that every tree has a life pattern and is not merely a mechanical reaction to the environment."[43]

Today, Adler would see a myriad of environments fostering the freedom of lifestyles, some excessive, which have left us with a global epidemic of obesity or *Globesity*.

From a millionaire's to green living, a lifestyle is how we choose to live, and it consists of attitudes, values, cultures and decisions.

---

[43] http://webspace.ship.edu/cgboer/adler.html

When others see our lifestyles, they observe conduct—mostly habits, behaviors and actions. In today's world, our lifestyle has become our sense of identity, so closely are we tied to movements like being politically correct, going green or identifying with a generation like Boomers, Gen X or Gen Y.

Healthy Means Lively

This section offers you the perfect opportunity to learn about and plan for a healthier lifestyle that can include appropriate food, exercise, nutrition and balance.

This may need some re-evaluation and prioritization on your part based upon your answers to the following questions.

• **Are you overweight or obese?** Which category you might fit in depends upon the amount of fat you carry. On the Body-Mass Index you would be overweight with a body mass index between 25 and 29.9. If your BMI is 30 or above, you are obese on that scale.

• **Do you have a high percentage of fat to muscle ratio?** Note that bodybuilders or athletes may have a high body mass range because of their high percentage of muscle. But a woman who is ten to fifteen pounds overweight and in the 30th percentile range for fat, needs an exercise discipline as much as someone whose fat ratios are bulging through their clothes. The reason is simple: fat cells produce an overload of leptin, which derails the feeling of fullness when eating. We eat more, and cause more hormonal miscues.

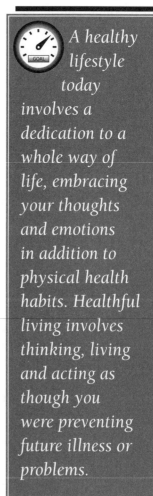

A healthy lifestyle today involves a dedication to a whole way of life, embracing your thoughts and emotions in addition to physical health habits. Healthful living involves thinking, living and acting as though you were preventing future illness or problems.

> *Obese people and you have the same number of fat cells; the difference is the size of these fat cells. You don't become overweight because you make more fat cells, but the fat globules swell each fat cell and increase your body size.*

• **Do you have inflammation?** Mounting evidence supports exercising to reduce inflammation.[44] In a recent article in *Scientific American* magazine, the writer examined the benefits of exercise from a number of studies. One benefit was reduced inflammation, especially associated with heart problems.[45]

• **Have a too-busy or excessive sedentary lifestyle?** Let's face it…the pounds creep on when we are so busy that we don't eat right or slow down. Worry and stress produce that hormone cortisol, which contributes to weight gain.

> *Cortisol affects you whether you are busy or sedentary.*

• **Do you know that you can start very slowly?** If you are new to the exercise scene, then the following pages will help you start moving gently, first to increase your energy, and then to choose how to exercise for your weight and energy levels.

• **Do you know which exercise is best for you?** We've read about the need for strength training, calorie burning and cardiovascular workouts. We need a bit of each, and how we achieve that depends upon our level of vitality and energy.

---

[44] Ford, E.S. "Does exercise reduce inflammation? Physical activity and C-Reactive protein among US adults." Epidemiology, (2002) Sept; 13(5) pp561-8.

[45] Ballantyne, C. "Does exercise really make you healthier? We examine five claims about the benefits of weight lifting and aerobics which carry the most…weight." Scientific American. January 2, 2009.

> **DOCTOR TAI'S IMPORTANT TIP**
>
> *You have to start with an exercise that you enjoy and that aligns with your goals for weight loss.* **The key is to move daily.**

• **Consider yourself a stressed or burned out person?** When stressed, we might feel rushed, be forgetful, or wake up in the middle of the night thinking about something. Although you're stressed, you are still engaged in life, even if adrenalin runs you for brief periods. You are moving to burnout when you feel exhausted and want to disengage from life.

When you believe stress is now a chronic factor in your life, you need exercise to move past the fatigue or other symptoms set in.

• **Are you meeting the goals you've set for yourself?** When you reshape your body, you also reconfigure your self worth... your image and feeling about yourself. So each goal you set counts, in so far as it is realistic for you, and you can achieve in small steps.

☞ *Achieving five minutes on the treadmill does wonders for feeling great about yourself. The joy of goal setting is that there is no failure. Each day you take the first step again, and again...you work wonders!*

Decision Is A Final Choice

Steven G. Aldana, expert on lifestyle choices, shows in his book *The Culprit and The Cure* that good choices can add ten to twenty years to our life spans. **The choices he cites as most important are diets and exercise,** to which we devote complete chapters to provide accurate and scientific information.

Making a decision is to come to a resolution after looking at all the choices. Think of a decision as your **final choice.** For example, you choose walking as your daily exercise, and you also decide that you will do it faithfully three times a week. Or, you may choose not to eat a certain food at any given time because of its calories.

 A firm decision to never eat it deletes that food from the buffet of your mind. The food no longer tempts you.

Out of Sight, Out of Mind

Jada was twenty-five pounds overweight and had to make some hard decisions about her diet. For example, she had low-fat yogurt for breakfast every morning. Each afternoon at work, she ate one cookie with her coffee. Her lunches and dinners were well planned in a healthy format, and she walked three times a week. Her decision was to toss the cookies from her kitchen cabinets and her office desk. She explained her thinking, "When I know the cookies are available, I think about it and I want to eat it right away. If I cut out the cookies from my snack time and don't buy them, cookies cease to exist for me. Out of sight, out mind and out of mouth. That is a decision, and a final one at that!"

 You'll need the savvy and competence to make solid decisions about food and exercise to re-establish a healthy lifestyle. Right eating and exercising are no longer just options in your life; it's mandatory. They are life-affirming decisions that demand your strength of will.

One woman, whom I'll call Sandra, is a 52-year old participant of the Bauhinia study. Sandra said that she liked to see immediate gratification of seeing results quickly to stay motivated on a diet. Who can blame her?

She noticed that after menopause, she could easily gain five pounds in a weekend if on vacation or visiting a friend. Her waistline thickened. In the evening, she was prone to salt or sugar cravings.

Bauhinia, in the form of **The Thin Factors** vanished the night cravings. Over the course of the study, she went down two dress sizes, and is still counting. Sandra had been a veteran dieter who tried other supplements, to no avail except side effects like skin breakouts and "feeling speedy." Sandra felt no side effects from bauhinia.

In fact, researchers questioned all subjects about any side effects with **The Thin Factors**. The positive side effects were having more energy, feeling lighter, and a general feeling of well-being.

Two foundations of a healthy lifestyle are getting enough sleep and regularly managing stressors through an easy strategy of deep breathing technique.

Chapter Sixteen
SLEEP WELL & BREATHE EASY

To insure good health: eat lightly, breathe deeply,
live moderately, cultivate cheerfulness,
and maintain an interest in life.
William Londen

What Is Normal Sleep?

There are two types of sleep. The first is called REM for rapid eye movement. REM is an active sleep in which your eyes move rapidly back and forth, and the body below the neck is still because the nerve impulses down the spinal cord are blocked. This is the sleep of dreams.

The second type of sleep is NREM or non-REM sleep, which has several stages from drowsiness through deep sleep. In the drowsy stage you wake easily and may feel you haven't slept. In deeper stages, you may feel like you cannot wake up and feel disoriented.

Since we sleep for one-third of our lives, how sleep helps us is often misunderstood, especially with respect to our hormones. Sleep provides the brain and body's restoration, especially during non-REM sleep.

• Disrupted sleep equals hormone dis-regulation. For example, the stress hormone cortisol is higher and growth hormone declines under these conditions.

• Anabolic hormones like growth hormone and DHEA, which are secreted in our growth years through our mid-twenties, rise during the non REM sleep phases.

• As we age, we spend less time in non-REM sleep.

• Disrupted sleep produces anxiety, fatigue, and cognition problems like recall difficulty or problem solving.

Knowing the problems that come from lack of sleep encourages us to crawl under cozy blankets with a good book and a set time for lights out.

DOCTOR TAI'S IMPORTANT TIP

Our hormone secretions rise and fall according to an internal timer. Setting and maintaining a regular schedule for sleep for our hormones is a first, simple and powerful strategy for a weight loss program since they regulate or mood and resilience.

The 8-Hour Rule!

The traditional notion that a person needs a good eight to ten hours of sleep at night holds true, even in the face of the Internet and cable television providing twenty-four hour entertainment. Lack of sleep disrupts every physiologic operation in the body, just as an adequate amount of sleep allows our bodies to restore and balance them.

Research has shown that decreased sleep leads to a larger appetite and food cravings. The natural next result is overeating and, therefore, an Increase In fat storage.

One recent study reported a consistently increased risk of obesity among short sleepers in both children and adults. This cross-sectional study from around the world was inclusive of data on 604,509 adults (ages 15-102 years) and 30,002 children (ages 2 to 12). [46]

---

[46] Cappuccio, F.P. MD et. al. "Meta-analysis of Short Sleep Duration and Obesity in Children and Adults" Journal of Sleep (05-01-08).

Link Between Sleep Deprivation and Obesity

Earlier studies have documented that **sleep-deprived adults produced more of the stomach's ghrelin, a hormone that promotes hunger, and less leptin, the hormone that signals fullness.** This same pattern of sleep deprivation and hunger appears to also affect babies and toddlers studied in a Harvard research project.

Babies and toddlers who slept less than 12 hours a day were at greater risk for being overweight in preschool. Viewing television heightened the affect.[47]

"Another interesting correlation between obesity and sleep disorders occurs in the body's inflammatory response. Obesity is associated with increased levels of pro-inflammatory cytokines (proteins produced by white blood cells that act as chemical messengers between cells)," reported Alexandro N. Vgontzas, MD, ScD, director of the Center for Sleep Disorder Medicine at the Department of Psychiatry, Pennsylvania State University's Milton S. Hershey Medical Center in Hershey.[48]

In addition, other prevalent hormonal contributions to weight gain are the stress hormones cortisol and orexin, a peptide hormone produced by nerve cells in the hypothalamus that stimulates eating.

DOCTOR TAI'S IMPORTANT TIP

We now know that persons, who sleep for shorter hours, who are deprived of sleep or whose sleep is disrupted, increase their risk of being overweight. This holds true for infants, children, teens and adults. The following are recommended hours of sleep for maintaining hormonal balance and health.

Infants and babies need sleep for 15 hours.

---

[47] Taveras, E. M. et.al. "Short Sleep Duration in Infancy and Risk of Childhood Overweight." Ped

[48] Kauffman, L. "Could Sleep Loss Cause Obesity?" Sleep Review Journal (July-August, 2006)

Toddlers' sleep patterns shift to 12 to 14 hours.

Preschool children need 11 to 13 hours.

Adolescents need 9 hours a night.

Adults need 7 to 8 hours a night.

Individualize Your Sleep Program

Remember those are general recommendations. Unless you fall right into the general classification, you really need to customize your sleep requirements. To individualize, you'll have to find out how many hours you would ordinarily sleep without the assistance of an alarm clock.

In other words, sleep until you wake up naturally on the average over a period of 7 days. That is your normal sleeping pattern and shows how many hours of sleep your body needs. If you need to wake up one hour earlier, then adjust your sleeping pattern easily by going to bed one hour earlier.

Another way to individualize your sleeping program is to always go to bed at the same time every night to maintain a consistent habit that is sustainable. The human body loves predictable consistency, especially when it comes to sleep.

Breathing Basics

The most basic movement of energy within the brain and body is the flow of oxygen through breathing.

Westerners are known for their shallow breathing, that is, chest or thoracic breathing. This stressful breathing pattern is worse if you are overweight or obese because of restricted airflow and pressure on the diaphragm.

The first, most important exercise is the simplest…to breathe into the abdomen, and it may require some breath retraining. As Gabriel Cousens, MD stated, "At least ninety percent of our metabolic energy should come from our breathing."

The benefits of proper breathing are so healthful.
  • **Enhances metabolism**
  • **Burns calories**
  • **Starts the thermogenic process**
  • **Energizes you**

Breathing Into The Abdomen

According to Tom Goode, ND, founder of the International Breath Institute,[49] breathing into the abdomen is best started and practiced in a reclining position so you feel the movement of your abdomen. When comfortable with the process, you can do abdominal breathing when watching television, walking your dog or standing at the sink.

DOCTOR TAI'S IMPORTANT TIP

Place one hand on the abdomen below the navel and the other on the chest. As you inhale in a slow count to four, breathe into and expand the abdomen, as if you were filling a balloon.

Stretch and extend the lower belly, and then exhale fully. The chest does not move at all. Continue breathing with minimal pause between inhale and exhale. All of the emphasis is upon your inhale. The exhale is a release of the tension created during your inhale.

[49] Goode, Thomas, ND. Breathe & Grow Rich (Dallas, Texas: Inspired Living International, 2008)

So you will inhale and relax...inhale...and relax. Close your eyes as you are breathing and then be still for a few minutes when you are done. Allow your breathing to normalize before continuing with your activities.

If you practice this simple breathing pattern several times a day, every day, for five or ten minutes, you will lower your blood pressure, experience the relaxation response, and feel more alert and energized.[50] Eventually, you can use this same breath to raise metabolism while walking or watching television. Do it for ten minutes or longer, and you also detoxify the body by increasing the lymph flow and movement.

> ### *Breathing and Holding*
> *Once you feel comfortable with deeper, effective breathing, you can pair it with isometrics and strengthen your core abdominal muscles. First inhale and expand the abdomen, then exhale completely and pull in the muscles. Hold the tension for five seconds and release. Rest and repeat while eventually extending the taut holding pattern from five to ten seconds.*

Family Considerations
Our eating and sleep patterns tend to conform to the lifestyle of the family. Here are some factors for you to consider when setting schedules for you and your children.

Studies on Children's Television & Obesity
One study in the *Archives of Pediatrics & Adolescent Medicine* looked at the relationships between watching television, energy intake, physical activity and obesity in boys and girls who were 8 to 16 years old.

---

[50] www.InternationalBreathInstitute.com

Obesity rates were lowest among children watching one-hour or less of television; and was highest among those watching four hours or more a day.[51]

Another longitudinal study stated that television watching was an independent predictor of the change in the child's body-mass index, triceps and the sum of the five skin folds throughout childhood. In short, the children between four and eight who watched the most television during childhood had the greatest increase in body fat over time.[52]

In summary, children who watch a lot of television are likely to
- **Have lower grades in school**
- **Be less drawn to reading**
- **Exercise less**
- **Be overweight**

---

[51] Carlos, J. et. al. Television Watching, Energy intake, and Obesity in US Children. Arch Pediatr Adolesc Med. 2001;155:360-365.

[52] Proctor, M.H. Television viewing and change in body ft from preschool to early adolescence: The Framingham Children's Study. International Journal of Obesity (2003) 27, 827–833. doi:10.1038/sj.ijo.0802294

DOCTOR TAI'S IMPORTANT TIP

Controlling Television Time

Television can provide educational entertainment if your child views a program, not television. Follow these guidelines for television watching:

Ages 0 to 2 years – no television

Ages 3 to 5 years – watch special programs up to one hour a day, or an educational hour extended what the child learned into books or activities that enhance language, motor skills and play time.

School-age children - Parents of school age children should have time restrictions not just for television (suggested up to four hours), but also for your child's immersion into the electronic world that includes Ipod, Nintendo, X-box activities and time on the computer. Children and parents can determine how time is spent in educational work, leisure activities, peer activities and entertainment.

Chapter Seventeen

THE GOAL IS FITNESS

If we eat less fat, why are we fatter?

Fat Ratio?

What exactly is too much fat? Becca, a fifty-five-year old woman who stood at five feet, eight inches, was proud that she had kept her slender, 130-pound figure throughout her adulthood. She had never exercised much, but she knew that she had to start at her age for health benefits and to maintain her high energy levels. She went to an exercise studio with a thirty-minute exercise program designed for women. She was astounded to find out from the trainer, who measured her fat ratio that she was in the 90th percentile for fat versus muscle. Becca thought she was in good health, but discovered she was not fit, and her doctor would consider her fat-to-muscle ratio as not healthy.

This is a fairly common problem. People with over 10% body fat, even when they eat right and feel in good health, may not be fit.

Our level of fitness is an important predictor of mortality.

Fit Ratio

Health fitness is what we seek in our weight loss programs for that includes physical fitness, emotional and mental fitness. Fitness encompasses the topic of body fat in comparison to body weight.

Fitness means having the ability to perform physical activity with the energy and strength to feel good.

In sport's circles, our body composition is lean mass versus fat.

A recent study found that one's waist-to-hip ratio was a better indicator of future heart problems than the body-mass-index.[53]

The rationale for the measurement of waist circumference is the accumulated fat in the belly, where the white fat spews out inflammation, which is associated positively with increased risk for type 2 diabetes, high blood pressure and heart health issues.

We don't realize how at risk we are for inflammation and toxicity, especially if we have gained even a mild ten pounds around the middle. Like Becca, men and women may live active lives, but they are not active in the right ways by walking or exercising consistently to burn calories or fat.

DOCTOR TAI'S IMPORTANT TIP

I've been asked all of the *basic weight loss* **questions:**

Don't I have to burn calories? Should I start a running program?

Where do I start?

Your weight loss program starts with movement and exercise, which we cover in the next chapter.

Begin now with integrating abdominal breathing into your daily routine. That will spark the thermogenic effect.

Take a daily dose of **The Thin Factors** *bauhinia support to help your appetite control biochemistry and thoroughly clean the satiety receptors.*

Take **Craving Factor** *to clean and rejuvenate your gut and*

---

[53] Elevated waist-hip ratio, not high body mass index, is associated with a greater risk of death" - American Journal of Clinical Nutrition, August 2006; 84:449-460.

*stomach to stop cravings born from gut to brain hormone signal disruption and **Max Slim** to kick up the resting metabolism so your body burns the extra calories, moving the body away from starvation or famine mode.*

Slimming liposome *cream applied to the fat areas of the tummy and thighs will thermogenically melt and reduce the fat.*

Know what a calorie is and understand why it counts.

Get rid of the sugar and bring Stevia into your home.

Plan your exercise program as you move through the next chapter.

Plan your menus and food decisions carefully and deliberately.

Keep a food diary. Research showed that a method of feedback to be highly beneficial. This has proven to be absolutely essential for us to know with certainty where we went right and where exactly we went wrong.

What Is A Calorie?

Calorie has an official definition and also the one we give it in reference to eating and exercising. Officially, calorie is the measurement of heat needed to raise the temperature of one liter of water by one degree.

 Unofficially, calories measure the energy contained in food and beverages we ingest. They are found in fat, carbs, protein and alcohol.

Basically calories are a measure of our body's fuel. In the body, the excess calories are stored as fat.

👉 *Each of us has a basic level of caloric daily need that fuels the energy that keeps the body running and performing our chores.*

👉 *Excess calories we eat turn to fat when they are not burned or when we are not active enough through work or exercise.*
**Movement and activity burn calories.
We'll gain about one pound for every 3500 calories in excess and over our bodies' needs.**

• The USDA recommends a caloric intake of 2000 calories for the average American to maintain weight. The caloric intake suggested for losing weight is 1200 to 1500 calories a day.

• One gram of protein has about four calories and has a higher metabolic burn rate. One gram of fat has about nine calories, and one gram of carbohydrate has about four calories, but a lower metabolic burn rate than protein.

In the diet chapter, you will understand how to eat appropriately for your calorie count and glycemic food intake.

Start to Build Energy
One basic truth about our human body is that we are designed to work, and if we don't move our bodies, we lose the ability to be flexible, active, energetic and vital.

Movement and exercise are essential for the thermogenesis activity, the imperative key to turn up

our body temperature and burn off excess calories.

An additional benefit is improvement in circulation and removal of toxic by-products that I've mentioned several times. The positive effects of movement are oxygen intake through consistent deeper breathing, increase in muscle mass, and burning calories faster.

Exercise increases bone density, which makes movement a healthful activity for all men and women who are in their forties or older.

Movement works with emotional energy, burning away negative moods, just like it burns fat. Our children, then, also benefit immensely from movement, just like their parents and grandparents. Exercise is the absolute foundation for any successful weight loss program.

It takes ten to twelve weeks of consistent exercise to become fit. It only takes one session of deep, abdominal breathing or fifteen minutes of brisk walking to feel better and improve your health and move consistently toward your goal of being fit and healthy.

Chapter Eighteen

EXERCISES FOR ENERGY & FLEXIBILITY

The first time I see a jogger smiling, I'll consider it.
Joan Rivers

Previous chapters showed that any exercise program, especially if you are overweight or obese, must start with the basics of breathing and movement. Movement serves twin purposes of getting energy flowing through you and strengthening your core.

If you don't move, you stagnate and set the stage for diseases. Remaining flexible and mobile is done mostly through stretching and walking.

This chapter discusses flexibility and stretching and other gentle aspects of movement to help you gain strength and vitality. They increase mobility, flexibility, stability, and strength and turn on muscles that you haven't used. These suggestions are beginner's exercises. With further education, you can extend and amplify the same movements into other broader exercise patterns.

Stretches
• Standing erect, stretch the left arm behind your neck and touch your spine. Use the right hand to pull the elbow toward your face while you resist and hold the tension for 10 seconds.

Do the same with the other arm. Repeat three times.

• Bend left knee behind you and hold it steady with your left hand. Balance and extend your right arm forward. Shift to the right hand and holding right foot and extend left hand. Hold the tension for ten seconds and then repeat the alternate stretching five times. If this is difficult, then start easy by pushing against a wall for balance and tension.

• Turn your face to the right, with your right palm, hold your chin in place and resist while your faces pushes against the palm and holds the tension for ten seconds. Repeat three times on the same side. Next do the same as your turn your head to the left.

• If you can handle the weight, stand on your toes, lifting gently up and down five times. Then rest. Repeat this exercise several times throughout your day, and include it in a regular stretching routine.

• Also hold you arms in front of you and lift your wrist, stretching hands and fingers for five seconds. Repeat three times.

• Standing with spine straight, lift your shoulders, scrunch your neck and hold tight for five seconds at a time. Repeat five times.

• Next, lift your arms above your head, interlace your fingers, palms upward and stretch and push upward, five seconds holding, and release. Repeat three to five times depending on your comfort level.

• With your arms still outstretched and fingers interlaced, push outward, to your left, to your right, and in front. Repeat three times and hold the tension as your stretch with a relaxation moment in between each push.

• Standing straight, legs slightly apart, rotate to the left, and then the right. Before each rotation, facing front, breathe into your abdomen, release your breath and hold muscles tight, and then rotate. Back to center, repeat breath and rotate to the opposite side.

• Holding the same posture and bending forward or back, even slightly, offer flexibility for your abdominal muscles.

Tai Chi

If you haven't yet heard of Tai Chi (tie-chee), then read on for this is a system for building energy, strength and flexibility that you will enjoy.

DOCTOR TAI'S IMPORTANT TIP

Tai Chi is an early form of martial arts training in China, and in the West, people practice the gentle movements as a meditative exercise. A session can last from thirty to sixty minutes, depending upon your capability. Tai Chi consists of a series of sets, and each set is a sequence of non-strenuous movements, which promotes circulation. What you might enjoy more are the relaxing benefits of well being after a session.

The feet remain rooted in the same position, while the torso and arms make graceful movements. These movements ease stress and help you relax. One learns Tai Chi by taking a class in your community or by following a Tai Chi video in your home.

Since Tai Chi arrived in the United States, research does support the health benefits for all, and especially those with balance issues or risks associated with obesity like high blood pressure, insulin resistance, breathing disorders and stress.

• In one study at Emory University, older persons participating in a fifteen-week course lowered their risk of falling by 47.5 percent.[54]

• According to several studies conducted by the Johns Hopkins University School of Medicine, tai chi reduced blood pressure, eased hypertension and improved cardiac health.[55]

[54] Wolf, Steven, L. PhD. "Tai Chi—An Innovative Approach to Reduce Falling in the Elderly." J Am Geriatric Soc (May, 1996).

[55] Derrick, Rachel Christmas. "Ease Hypertension with Tai Chi." Essence Magazine. Sept. 1998.

• Research from the University of Southern California showed that regular tai chi classes reduced lower back pain. In 50 volunteers between ages 18 and 65, with daily back pain, the pain decreased in half the people.[56]

Walking

Does walking cause weight loss? No one is really sure. However, I believe brisk walking and achieving a mild sweat is a phenomenal place to start and has a definite place in your weight loss program.

If you are in pain, suffer from joint or muscle pain, then participate in a regular exercise program like the older adults who decreased their disability risk and increased their likelihood for independence in one study at the University of Georgia.[57] Daily walking benefits are best realized at twenty minutes, increasing to thirty and maintaining that minimum at a casual pace.

> *Most people don't think of slow, meditative movements like Tai Chi or casual walking as exercises for burning calories. Not only do they release stress, but the simple act of moving can alleviate depression and anxiety.*

Benefits of Walking

- Adaptable to individual fitness levels
- Maintains the body's need for movement
- Supports time with friend or family
- Strengthens bones
- Uses almost as many calories as jogging
- Reduces risk of heart problems and diabetes
- Lowers blood pressure
- Enhances stamina
- Help the joints be flexible
- Decreases waist circumference

[56] Li, F., Harmer, P., McAuley, E. "Tai Chi Improves Physical Function in Sedentary Older Adults." Geriatrics. July 2000.

[57] University of Georgia (2008, July 22). Regular Walking Nearly Halves Elderly Disability Risk. ScienceDaily. Retrieved December 26, 2008.

Chapter Nineteen
EAGER TO EXERCISE

Exercise Planning

To accomplish exercise in our busy lives means we absolutely have to put it on our calendar.

From today forward, exercise becomes part of our scheduled activities along with brushing teeth, buying groceries, and taking the kids to their lessons.

> *From this day forward, feel the joy every morning when you say and hear this phrase, "I so value myself and my health that I am exercising today."*

Being overweight or obese means we'll choose functional exercises that get movement of energy started. Once we start exercises, the lactic acid clearing from muscles may feel achy.

You may think or are afraid that all exercise has to be hard, intense or painful. Not true! Exercise of

DOCTOR TAI'S IMPORTANT TIP

Add anti-inflammatory herbs from **MaxPain Specialist** (ginger oil, C. Yahusu, P.Lactifora, A. Sinensis, S. Arbor, A. Deharica) to your bauhinia and fresh, filtered water or natural brewed tea as part of your healthy lifestyle and you are good to go!

moderate intensity works as well as high-intensity exercise in reducing the risk of heart disease.[58]

> Our goals are to start slowly with abdominal breathing to fuel the metabolism, next commit to movement of some kind, like brisk walking for 30 minutes daily. Then move to functional exercises like Yoga or Pilates.

Functional Exercises

The term *functional exercise comes* from rehabilitation training, in which an exercise served the function or task in a person's life. For someone who needed muscle strength for lifting, then strength building was used.

DOCTOR TAI'S IMPORTANT TIP

A functional exercise for your movement might be to dance to music with a light rhythm for 30 minutes or more. The need for endurance could involve slowly going up and down half a flight of stairs twice. Muscle building could be lifting a two-pound or five-pound weight in each hand as you watch television. Igniting the metabolism might be three ten-minute daily breaks for deeper, more effective breathing.

Think about your day and list what actions you take: Lifting groceries, walking, putting dishes away, standing at the stove, playing with children, pushing a stroller, lifting cat litter bags or dog food boxes or bags, sitting at a desk or on a couch. Let's get innovative about what you can do.

---

[58] Manson J. E, et. al. "A Prospective Study of Walking as Compared with Vigorous Exercise in the Prevention of Coronary Heart Disease in Women. New Engl J Med 341: 650-658, 1999.

Reaching up: Put a glass away, and stretch both arms high into the air and breathe into the abdomen, tightening the muscles on the exhale. Relax and repeat.

Pushing: If you stand in the kitchen while food cooks, place your hands on the kitchen counter, then lean into the counter and move your feet back. Do five to ten counter push-ups at a time.

Squats: To strengthen knees and buttocks muscles, stand facing the counter or the back of a chair at arm's length. Squat only as far as is comfortable, keeping tush taut and out, and knees over the toes. Repeat five times, adding one more squat a day until you feel you are getting a good workout.

Simple Isometrics: Use a towel the size of a hand towel. Standing or sitting with your back straight, place the towel behind your neck, pulling it forward with both hands while your neck resists. Using the same towel, move it to the forehead and pull it taut for five seconds while resisting, then relax, and repeat five more times.

Walking in place: While watching television, stand and march in place, lifting knees to a comfortable height. Walk for two minutes, rest for one, walk for two. Continue this each evening, adding one minute to your marching time every third day.

DOCTOR TAI'S IMPORTANT TIP

Always pace yourself to do what is enjoyable and comfortable, the key is to achieve a slight moist sweat and maintain that higher temperature of exercise for as long as you like. The purpose is not seeing how hard you can push yourself. Rather, how long can you sustain a comfortable pace and still be willing to do it again tomorrow, and again and again? If you try too hard and kill yourself in this heroic effort, you certainly won't do yourself any good and for sure, you won't want to do it again tomorrow.

Interval Exercising

A study from the University of Wisconsin-Oshkosh, in the October 2001 issue of the *Journal of the American College of Nutrition*[59] showed that three 10-minute bouts of exercise, or two 15-minute bouts, and one 30-minute bout were each equally effective in increasing aerobic capacity and reducing body fat. The exercise was paired with a restricted calorie diet for those in the study.

Short bouts of intense exercise are called "interval exercises" or training, 2 minutes of maximum, fast-paced exercise followed by 8 minutes of slower comfortable exercise, and it is perfect for those beginning a new program. It ignites metabolism quicker by burning energy stored in muscles in the form of glucagon to fuel short bursts of energy. It also creates lactic acid as a byproduct and causes that achy, used-up feeling.

Short bursts of interval exercise might look like any combination of time elements adding up a thirty-minute workout daily.
- Five six-minute sessions
- Three ten-minute sessions
- Two fifteen-minute sessions
- One thirty-minute sessions

For example, Tom walks his dog each morning several times around the block. He is a spry walker and wanted to incorporate interval training into his morning walks. After speaking with a fitness trainer as to his best options, he incorporated three minutes of jogging or speed walking and then eight minutes of lively walking. His daily exercise routine takes between 30 to 45 minutes. His Great Dane also enjoys the activities.

[59] Schmidt, W. D. et/ al. "Effects of Long versus Short Bout Exercise on Fitness and Weight Loss in Overweight Females." J. Am. Coll. Nutr. 20: 494-501

> ### Benefits
> *Don't be discouraged if you don't see weight loss immediately. Have faith in your body, which loses visceral fat first. On the inside, that fat peels off like onions, layer by layer.*

The "interval exercising" works in your behalf by
- **Burning more calories**
- **Improves insulin receptivity**
- **Enables you to sleep soundly**
- **Builds cardio-vascular fitness, allowing you to exercise longer as you gain strength and endurance**
- **Improves breathing capacity and ability.**

Rev It Up...

If you are ready to rev up your engine and move to a more intense or prolonged workout, consider the treadmill first. Although some people consider the treadmill boring, with exercising music and an optimistic attitude, short bursts with intensity are extremely beneficial to you health.

New research shows that aerobic exercise (intended to improve cardio) like a 60-minute workout on the treadmill, caused ghrelin, which promotes appetite, to drop and peptide YY to increase.

"The finding that **hunger is suppressed** during and immediately after vigorous treadmill running is consistent with previous studies showing that strenuous aerobic exercise transiently **suppresses appetite**," reported David Stensel, senior author of the research.[60]

Revving up your metabolism certainly burns more calories. Insure you ease yourself into a program over months, increasing vitality and continuing to breathe deeply as you move from movement and stretching to walking, then to low and eventually high intensity programs for interval exercising.

---

[60] Broom et al. The influence of resistance and aerobic exercise on hunger, circulating levels of acylated ghrelin and peptide YY in healthy males. AJP Regulatory Integrative and Comparative Physiology, 2008.

Chapter Twenty

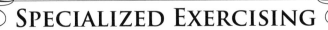

SPECIALIZED EXERCISING

While fitness is our goal, the exercise programs in this section are for weight loss. Eating right and exercise are partners in this endeavor. We must do both to achieve our results.

> *For a program to work, I advise that first you determine your caloric needs and focus on creating a calorie deficit each day. Strength or resistance training, which challenges muscles, preserves your muscle tissue. Interval cardio training partners with resistance, even at levels of low challenge or intensity. More importantly, do what you enjoy with a passion for your health, appearance, and optimism.*

Activity Awareness

Being aware of activities every day means you are always on the lookout for pushing the edge. Being aware means you have health on your mind and seek each day to improve your metabolism. You take every opportunity to stay active. In addition, you train your brain and body to go the extra mile. Maybe you…

- Drink fresh water or iced tea instead of snacking.

- Climb stairs when you can.

- Park at the far end of a grocery store's parking lot, and then walk to the store.

- Use your television watching time to be productive regarding exercise (waking in place or on the treadmill; lifting light weights, alternating arms as you sit; using the hand towel for simple resistance exercises).

- Be on the treadmill, a stair master or stationary bicycle for short bursts of free time.

- Ride your bicycle around the neighborhood.

- Walk with your children.

• Garden with your grandchildren or a friend who shares your love of nature.

Awareness is also choosing the types of exercises you feel meet your need as you starting with breathing retraining, movement and then include specific exercise types to meet your fitness goals.

Know Your Core

Most people think of specific types of exercises for cardio and strength without considering the core or body center, which provides stability and makes it easier for you to exercise.

*The **CORE** of our bodies includes the trunk and pelvis and works the muscles of the lower back, pelvis, abdomen and hips.*

Think about how often you do tasks from this center like tie a shoe, pick up something from the floor, reach for an object, or swing a golf club, tennis racket or baseball bat.

Weak core muscles leave you with weak posture and possibly back pain.

If you are overweight or have poor core strength, the easiest place for you to start is with a fitness ball.

• Sit on the ball, spine straight and do the abdominal breathing in sets of three to five. Rest and bounce gently, then repeat the set.

• Keeping your back straight and toes or feet touching the floor, bounce gently.

• Standing with knees bent slightly for comfort, back straight and bent slightly forward, hold the ball between your hands and extend your arms. Stiffen and relax, repeat.

• In the same position with arms parallel to the floor, rotate to the left and right. Or lift the ball up, stiffen arms and relax, and repeat.

Cardiovascular Training

As the name implies, cardiovascular exercises strengthen heart and lungs, and the basic exercise is abdominal breathing. Cardio training is working the body to get oxygen and blood to the muscles. A higher heart rate burns more calories.

Interval exercises work best here. That means 2 minutes in extra fast pace and 8 minutes at a comfortable pace. For example, you can burn 100 calories in a low intensity exercise like walking or you can burn 160 calories in ten minutes of high intensity exercise.

 Remember, it is more about maintaining and consistency, how long can you keep a comfortable warm pace.

Ultimately, for a cardio workout for fat loss, you want to build up to a three sessions a week of twenty minutes. Five times a week is awesome! Be happy to start one day at a time, building slowly as you feel the body heat building and the heart pumping.

In a long-term study of fitness at the Cooper Aerobics Center in Dallas, Texas, more than 80,000 subjects followed over thirty years have demonstrated some solid facts. The ore fit subjects have heart-disease death rates 50 percent lower than the least fit. They are also less likely to have strokes, develop diabetes, lower cancer rates and lower risk for senility or dementia.[61] Of most interest to us is the showing "**that fit-but-fat are nearly as healthy as the fit-of-normal-weight**". Regular exercise offsets the dangers of being overweight."[62]

DOCTOR TAI'S IMPORTANT TIP

Here are general guidelines for **cardio training specifically for weight loss**. For endurance and cardio workouts, apply the concept to walking uphill, walking stairs, cycling, hitting a punching bag, working on an elliptical machine or treadmill.

Do cardio training in the morning on an empty stomach to pull the energy from the muscles and burn the sugar. The next best time is after weight training.

Memorize this truth! Your body won't burn any fat until it has finished burning sugar first. That's right, the secret to burning fat is the sequence the body goes through...first it burns the stored sugar off the muscle, then it moves to burning the excess sugar stored in the liver. Only after those sugars are gone, will the body start burning fat around the body.

So the lesson to be learned is this: go nice and steady, achieving a moist sweat, and keep it going comfortably for as long as you enjoy it.

Then do it again.

When you set up this routine stick to it and **the result is magnificent!**

[61] Burfoot, A. "Grave Concerns." Runners World (11-25-2008) http://healthandfitness.sympatico.msn.ca/HealthyLiving/ContentPosting_RW?newsitemid=

[62] Ibid.

So, whatever you snack or eat turns to sugar and then goes back into the muscle and liver. Now you have to start all over again. Without exercise it takes **4 hours without eating to burn the sugar from the muscle and liver...only after that period of time does the body begins to burn the fat.**

So now you can think in terms of breakfast, lunch and dinner...what amount will you eat and when should you? Obviously the most promising time to lose weight is at night principally. If you don't eat after 8 PM until morning, you take advantage of this science to lose weight. THIS IS ALSO part of diet planning in the next chapter... when to eat and how much to eat. Of course the secret is when not to eat.

Be happy in the beginning of your cardiovascular training with the short bursts. Walking for three minutes and slowly building to six minutes and then ten is good for building endurance.

Later, use interval training for endurance, of 2 minutes at very fast pace followed by 8 minutes of a slower endurance pace. Building through walking, than an intense cycle, than an endurance cycle, and start again.

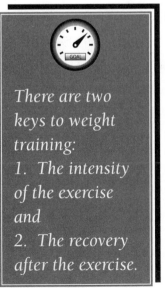

There are two keys to weight training:
1. The intensity of the exercise and
2. The recovery after the exercise.

Strength Training

What is the relationship of strengthening your body to weight loss?

Women need to strengthen muscles, as do men, especially in the menopausal or postmenopausal years. Women don't have the muscle mass to develop the curves men have. Yet, the benefits of women's strength trainings are increasing bone density, muscle mass and strength. For example, lifting a two-pound or a five-pound weight should be comfortable for eight to twelve repetitions. When the twelfth repetition feels too light, then you are ready for the next weight size.

To increase functional muscle size in the shortest amount of time, remember these words: infrequent, short, and intense. Research shows that muscles overcompensate up to a week after exercise and performing two to three exercises per session work for the average person.

For losing weight, lifting heavier weights for low repetition ranges is better than medium weights for longer repetition.

Exercise specialists suggest a full-body routine to include major muscle groups, which are back, chest, quads, shoulders, hamstrings and glutes, biceps, triceps, abs and calves.

Muscles burn more calories than fat! One pound of muscle burns around 45 calories each day while a pound of fat just sits there.

DOCTOR TAI'S IMPORTANT TIP

Think of muscle building activity as your weight loss friend. If you build just two pounds of muscle, it would, all by itself, burn off an extra pound of fat--each and every month.

Part V

BIO-HORMONES & TWO STAGE WEIGHT LOSS PROGRAM

Chapter Twenty-One

BIO-HORMONES & WEIGHT LOSS

Spectacular weight loss Program!

You can Look and feel fantastic!

They say...
> *It's not rocket science to lose weights: Burn more calories than you take in, you will lose weight! Easy, right?*

Not so to the majority of overweight people, middle aged, post menopausal women or andropausal men.

They say...

Most people think that people with weight problems because they do not exercise or discipline enough with their eating habits. I know you have all tried exercise, went on some types of diet programs that people have sworn by. You followed them faithfully but somehow, none of them worked for you. You felt hopeless that this was just the way you were going to look forever. You even started to psych yourself to thinking that you were not fat.. You were just a little round.... around the middle... the thighs...the butt...Oh! forget it!

The truth is, many women or men gain extra weight because of the normal demands of life... taking care of our children, household chores, running errands.... It all takes time and is all so draining. Who wants to come home after a full day of work, then drive the children around to their after school activities or help the children with their homework while cooking dinner, put children to sleep, and still have enough energy to go to the gym? This is madness! You are not superwoman or superman. We do what we need to do and then get ready for the next day.

Our bodies don't work like a robot. We do not have body parts that can be easily re-furbished and replaced. We are biological organisms that have complex systems of hormones, enzymes, and proteins. These intricate parts of our bodies help us cope with the hassles of life that surround us. Principally when it is post menopause or andropause, the body really goes downhill fast. I gain weight just smelling food!

How Do Bio-Hormones Effect you?

There is no one magic pill that can help you to lose weight in a week. If we are going to understand how our bodies work, we must start with the building blocks and how they work in our tissues to influence our health and weight loss.

> *The crucial hormones to understand concerning weight loss are thyroid, dehydroepiandrosterone (DHEA), cortisol, estrogen, Human Growth Hormone (HGH) and Human Chorionic Gonadotropin (HCG). When these hormones are out of balance or not functioning properly it is difficult and nearly impossible to control our weight.*

First, the thyroid gland produces **thyroid hormones** (T3 & T4) which regulate the metabolic rate, burning fat, and provide core temperature. They determine how well we burn calories in activity and **at rest**, how much of a problem we'll have with our weight. Thyroid hormones also regulate how our cells use oxygen and influence our growth and development. Abnormalities of the thyroid gland in producing hormones – either overproduction or underproduction – can result in adverse physical and energy effects. An overactive thyroid can result in heart palpitations, anxiety symptoms, diarrhea, and unsafe weight loss.

> *An underactive thyroid, as occurs in up to 50-60% of women and men over the age of 50, can result in **poor concentration, memory problems, feel cold most of the time, cold hands and feet, weight gain, thinning hair, low energy levels, feeling tired excessively, fatigue, muscle pain and weight gain.** If you have most of these symptoms, you may be suffering from low thyroid function.*

The second and third hormones **dehydroepiandrosterone (DHEA) and cortisol** are produced by the adrenal cortex. **DHEA - an anabolic or "building" hormone** - has "actor-like" characteristics. It is versatile, taking on a variety of roles at the same time by producing hormones and also converting them into other hormones.

A lack of DHEA has been linked to cancer, and animal studies have shown that DHEA supplementation helps prevent obesity, principally around the middle "bulging waist" and improves cognition. Many researchers believe that **DHEA improves glucose metabolism and may help protect against adult-onset diabetes.** Because DHEA is able to increase insulin sensitivity, it can improve the transport of glucose across cell membranes, specifically for improvement of energy and stamina and lowering the fatigue factor that ultimately helps to delay and improve the abnormal sugar metabolism of diabetes II.

Research has shown that one of the many extraordinary abilities of DHEA is that it restrains the negative effects of G6PDH, an enzyme known for its **"Fat Deposit"** factor. G6PDH turns glucose into fat cells; DHEA redirects the enzyme, turning it into **Energy** instead of fat.

In July 2003, *The Journal of Clinical Endocrinology and Metabolism* reported the findings of a Japanese research project. In the study, DHEA was given to 24 men with elevated cholesterol levels for 12 weeks. Each of the 24 men was given 25 mg of DHEA; a separate group received a placebo. The participants were assessed for endothelial (blood vessel) function, and blood samples were drawn to assess insulin sensitivity. The subjects who received the DHEA supplementation showed vasodilatation of the brachial arteries that increased significantly over the course of the course of 12 weeks, whereas the placebo group remained at base line levels. The Japanese researchers noted the subjects taking DHEA supplementation had a fasting plasma glucose level that was much lower, demonstrating increased insulin activity and receptor sensitivity. Blood vessel dysfunction (endothelium) causes vessels to become inflamed; therefore, **DHEA deficiency increases the potential to cause cardiovascular disease.** The researchers reported that the levels of age-related decline in DHEA are associated with a decrease of insulin sensitivity, which may cause Diabetes II.

We lose this "Youth Hormone" DHEA as we age. By the time we are 60 years old, we producing as much DHEA as we were under 10 years old.

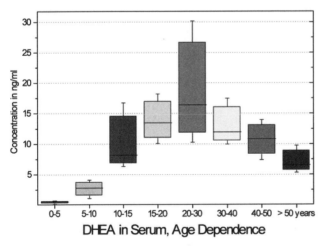

DHEA in Serum, Age Dependence

Of course, not only DHEA is affected, but also the **"Fat Burning" 7 Keto DHEA** goes down dramatically also. No wonder our fat cells do not know what to do! We just lost 75% of our fat burning capacity by our 60th birthday!

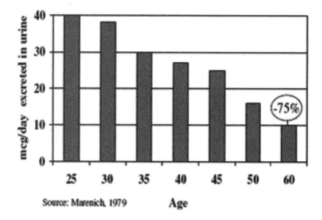

Source: Marenich, 1979   Age

Like DHEA, the hormone **Cortisol** is stimulated by the release of ACTH a 39-amino acid peptide that is produced by the anterior pituitary gland. Production of ACTH is in turn stimulated by corticotropin releasing hormone (CRH) released by neurons in the hypothalamus. CRH is released in a series of pulses that results in the rhythmic cycle secretion of ACTH and cortisol secretion. Only 3% to 10% of circulating cortisol is in the "free state" that is useable. Approximately 90% of cortisol is bound to corticosteroid-binding globulin that is produced mainly in the liver and has been found in all mammalian species. As is characteristic of most hormones, cortisol regulates the activity of the hypothalamic-pituitary-adrenal axis through its negative feedback effects on ACTH and CRH release.

Other functions of cortisol include maintaining glucose metabolism, regulation of blood pressure, and insulin release for blood sugar maintenance and dealing with stress, both physical and emotional. Unlike the other hormones, cortisol is a catabolic hormone, meaning that it breaks down enzymes and proteins to release energy.

An excess or a deficiency of cortisol is the primary cause of neurovascular and endocrine deterioration. **Cortisol excess causes tissues, proteins and muscles to continuously break down. Breaking down tissues, in turn, exhausts the adrenal cortex and increases the level of sugar in the bloodstream, depositing additional fat and causing**

accelerated aging. Cortisol's demands for higher insulin levels is very hard on the pancreas.

Hypersecretion of cortisol is associated with osteoporosis and undesirable fat distribution and swelling of the face as observed in Cushing's syndrome. The excess of cortisol depresses our immune system and increases vascular hypertension from water retention, thinning skin and thyroid destruction. On the other hand, hyposecretion of cortisol is associated with fatigue, inability to handle stress, mental confusion, symptoms of which include facial skin wrinkles, hyperpigmentation and muscle weakness, in other words, hyposecretion or severe lack of cortisol ages you really fast!!!

Finally, **Estrogen** is probably the most widely known and discussed of all hormones. Estrogen is produced in the ovaries, adrenal glands, and fat tissues. *The term "estrogen" includes a group of chemically similar hormones:* **Estrone (E1)**, **Estradiol** *(E2) (the most well known) and* **Estriol** *(E3) (the best known of all types of estrogen).* Estrogenic hormones are sometimes mistakenly referred to as exclusively female hormones when in fact both men and women produce them. The estrogenic hormones are uniquely responsible for the growth and development of female sexual characteristics and reproduction in both humans and animals.

Estrogen determines skeletal formation (wider hips), fat distribution (softer curves) and weight gain. Before high school (around the time when puberty strikes), girls are thin. After the age of 13, a physiological evolution usually takes place right before a person's eyes. Growth takes place, and girls turn into young ladies. Estrogen is the culprit in this caterpillar to butterfly transformation. Many girls can gain 20 to 30 pounds along with breast formation during puberty, which is also all accredited to estrogen. Not only are their complaints about weight gain, but menstrual cycles begin, which are usually accompanied by mood swings, water retention, and food cravings.

Every hormone has its good and its bad sides. Since women need estrogen it is reasonable to expect an estrogen deficiency to contribute to a woman's physical, mental, and emotional imbalance.

Estrogen has wide application throughout the body. For example, estrogen promotes formation of female secondary sex characteristics and excess estrogen, increases fat deposit in the stomach, butt and thighs. A diet of high fat increases level of estrogen and the incidence of breast cancer (*Ahlgrimm M. The HRT Solution. 1999; NY:A very Pub.*) In turn, the excess fat cells make more estrogen and the vicious cycle continues.

Estrone is produced by the ovaries and fat cells. The body fat in men and women also converts testosterone into estrone. Thus, the more fat one has, the more estrone is made.

Estrone, a characteristic of post-menopausal estrogen, serves as a reservoir the body can use for its primary form of estrogen since Estrone can be converted back into Estradiol. However, after menopause, excess body fat converts into Estrone. One method of dealing with this body fat is to balance natural hormones that will assist in the processing of this body fat into energy. **Progesterone** is the primary balance to excess estrogen and its negative effects of fat deposit, water retention, and mood swings. To decide which hormones to administer, we examine the natural bodily use of the natural bio-hormones and how the natural hormone, Human Chorionic Gonadotropin (HCG), might help us in our quest.

New Approach to Obesity - HCG
(Human Chorionic Gonadotropin)

Human Chorionic Gonadotropin is produced by the placenta in pregnancy to balance the body hormone and mobilize fat for energy. It stimulates both FSH and LH. Luteinizing hormones in women trigger ovulation and in men stimulate Leydig cell production of testosterone. These pituitary hormones LH (Luteinizing Hormone) are closely related to HCG in that all are glycosilated and have a dimeric structure comprising an Alpha and Beta chain. The amino acid sequences of the Alpha chain of all human glycoprotein hormones are nearly identical. Amino acid sequences of the beta subunits differ because of the unique immunological and biological activities of each glycoprotein hormone. Beta -HCG contains a carboxylic residue of 30 amino acids characteristic to HCG. **Because of the close structural similarity of HCG and LH, HCG can be used in a similar way as LH to increase lipolytic activity and in turn, increase the metabolic rate – which burns fat, principally bad fat around the waist and belly.**

HCG is often used as an LH substitute because it activates the same receptor, has a longer half life than LH, less costly, and the physiological use of HCG has no great risk of side effects. Evidence suggests that HCG promotes lipolytic activity (Fat burning activity). Since HCG does not mobilize in vitro lipids from the fat cell, it was hypothesized that the hypothalamic region might be the intermediate organ in HCG lipolytic action and energy production from its strong effects in perfectly balancing testosterone, DHEA, estrogen, and progesterone.

The HCG method includes patients' follow-up (daily visits to the doctor to be weighed), helping patients with their behavior modification program and control hunger factor and satiety. There are some similarities between the behavioral program included in the HCG protocol and a current behavior modification program for obesity treatment. **The 500 Kcal-diet as prescribed in the original treatment proved to be safe, easy tolerated, and effective.** Primary used in individual over 18 years old in both males and females, and hardly any contraindications to use the HCG method for the treatment of obesity. *Tolerance to the treatment is excellent, and many patients willingly request a second treatment without experiencing negative side effects.*

However, any Positive side effects are welcome! Such as beautiful silky skin, natural glow to the face, more energy and beautiful sculpting of fat away from waistline, hips, butt, and thigh.

Weight loss is safe and comfortable for patients, provided that they meticulously follow the prescribed diet **of no sugar, no oil, no fat, and low carbohydrates.** Any deviation from the protocol is apt to yield poor results. Even minor diet deviations may cause unwanted setbacks. But the results are fantastic if you don't deviate!

The HCG protocol is an appropriate approach to the treatment of obesity that also includes a behavior modification program as well as natural supplemental and dietetic aspects. ***When properly managed, the result is rapid weight loss of the Stage I and Stage II for a total of 70 days and improved body shape after treatment (Beautiful young body shape!).*** Clinical complications and unfavorable results are related to unsafe modifications of the protocol.

In the next chapter, we will discuss how the HCG protocol plus a change in accelerated fat burning metabolism is just the right combination to treat obesity.

> *A powerful combined procedure:* **HCG/Hunger Factor protocol plus natural supplements** *for the overweight body to overcome the resistance and burn the extra adipose tissue.*

Introduction

Adipose tissue (aka body fat) is found primarily underneath the skin (subcutaneous fat) and around the internal organs (visceral fat) or (Omentum fat), which act as signals to help communicate between outside and inside the cell. Fat cells membrane has specialized receptors. It has been a subject of great interest in recent years in obesity research because they carry the special signal to burn excess white fat cells.

Human fat cells possess both Alpha and Beta membrane adrenoreceptors, which affect adipose tissue metabolism differently. The major function of adrenoreceptors in white fat cells is to regulate the breakdown of triglycerides to free fatty acids and glycerol through lipolysis. Functions and mechanisms of action of adrenoreceptors in white fat cells are: A] Beta 1.2.3. receptors increase lipolysis rate; B] Alpha 2 receptors decrease lipolysis rate. An increase of Alpha activity is related to a decreased fat burn, whereas when you lose beta adrenergic activity you also decrease fat burn.

> *Abdominal adipocytes* (belly fat) are more responsive to the fat burning action of Beta-1 adrenergic agonists, while gluteal (butt fat) adipocytes are more resistant to fat burning action of Alpha-2-adrenergic agonists. Therefore, it is harder to lose those extra pounds of fat on the butt and thighs than of the stomach, and even harder when you are a woman.
>
> As you can see, Fasting also modifies the fat tissue burns. Fat around your belly is much less responsive to fasting diets. This may perpetuate the "pear shaped" obesity with enlarged waist.

We currently recommend using HCG Protocol (Stage I & II) plus the local application to the thigh area of a cream containing 7 keto-DHEA to stimulate extra fat cell melting capacity. This procedure is well accepted by patients with excellent results. No complications were reported with this combined method, and excellent research supports its conclusions. (See clinical reports)

7 Keto DHEA has 3 very effective "**Thermogenic**", meaning, Fat Burning pathways. The studies and research by Lardy in 1998 all shows excellent fat burning capacity of 7 Keto DHEA.

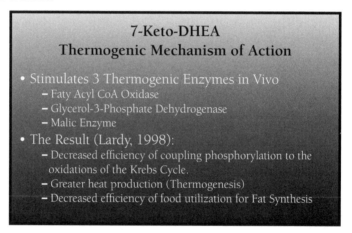

7 Keto DHEA research also show the natural biohormone 7 Keto increases the enzyme activity for greater Fat Burning capability in our body without stimulation or negative side effects.

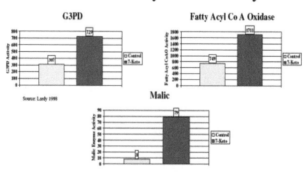

7-Keto significantly increased enzymatic activity vs. control group

2 clinical studies for weight loss versus placebo were performed "Random double blind placebo control trials"

(RDBPCT) for 8 weeks. The results were very significant favoring those subjects using 7 Keto DHEA supplements, they **lost more weight, lost more inches, lost more fat, lost more Body Mass Index, and increased Basal Metabolic Rate (BMR).**

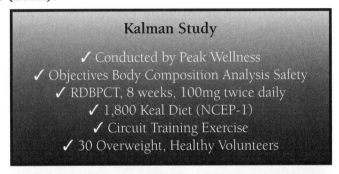

Kalman Study

✓ Conducted by Peak Wellness
✓ Objectives Body Composition Analysis Safety
✓ RDBPCT, 8 weeks, 100mg twice daily
✓ 1,800 Keal Diet (NCEP-1)
✓ Circuit Training Exercise
✓ 30 Overweight, Healthy Volunteers

Zenk Study

• Conducted by Minnesota Applied Research Center
• Objectives: Body Composition Analysis Safety
• RDBPCT, 8 weeks, 100mg Twice Daily
• 1,800 Keal Diet
• Cross-Training Exercises
• 35 Overweight, Healthy Volunteers

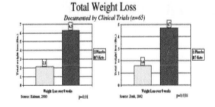

7-Keto produced 3 times more weight loss vs. placebo

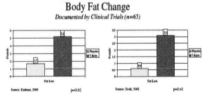

➢7-Keto produced 3 times more fat loss than placebo
➢80% of total weight loss was fat

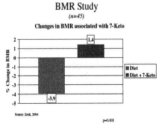

7-Keto significantly reduced BMI versus placebo

7-Keto increased BMR by 5.4% w/o Stimulants

Chapter Twenty-Two

GETTING STARTED

(Must complete Diet Program - Stage I First!)

1. If you are combining **HCG/Hunger Factor (Stage II Diet)** with other medications, you should discuss this with your physician.

2. **Pick your starting date.** If you are a menstruating woman, avoid starting the Stage II Diet protocol until after your period.

3. **Take "before" pictures from front, side and back profile.** Also, take measurements and record them on the "tracking our progress" form in this package. Determine your goal weight based on input from your physician and the appropriate weight chart.

4. Make sure you have the **prepared HCG/Hunger Factor and store it in the refrigerator** the day before your starting date.

5. On your starting date, begin taking HCG/ Hunger Factor (Stage II) at the **consistent time**, usually first thing in the morning.

6. The first two HCG/Hunger Factor days (Stage II) are your **"load" days**. These days should be spent eating as much fattening food as possible to restore structural fat and avoid hunger at startup.

7. Starting with the **3rd Hunger Factor day**, use the **500 Calorie Diet** and *continue until 72 hours after your Hunger Factor is finished, the minimum number of diet days for a cycle is 23 days with a maximum per cycle of 40 HCG/Hunger Factor days. **Note: You continue the 500 calorie diet for three days after the last dose of HCG/Hunger Factor.**

8. Enjoy your new body!

9. Weight adjustment is a **5 bottles of water** with Craving Factor throughout the day, one salad for AM & noon and for dinner, a large steak and salad, vegetable soups in between during the day, **no oil, no carb, no sugar** and continue **until you get back to your desired weight.**

Summary of a Typical Round

DIET PROGRAM - STAGE I

Prof. Dr. Paul Ling Tai's Scientific Comprehensive approach on Overweight and Obesity targets the 4 Essential problems of Weight Gain - **The 4 Resistances to Losing Weight!**

4 Resistances of Weight Loss & Obesity

1. **Leptin Resistance** – *Satiety Dysfunction, Overeating & Craving*
2. **Insulin resistance** – *Glucose Metabolism Abnormality*
3. **Adrenaline Resistance** – *Abnormal Glycogen Metabolism*
4. **Thyroid Resistance**– *Low resting metabolism Rate & Low Thermogenic*

Stage I of this Diet program is designed <u>to cleanse</u> and <u>prepare</u> the body and to <u>lose 5 to 10 lbs</u> in the first 30 days.

1200 calorie Diet – with special Supplements

The only way to lose weight is to burn more calories per day than you take in. But a good diet should also include foods you enjoy eating. If the calorie content of your diet menu is too low, your body will rebel and you may binge. If the calories are too many, you won't lose weight. Of course, we always recommend a good exercise program with your diet plan. Walking briskly 20 minutes a day will speed your weight loss progress. Don't forget to take your daily vitamins & minerals!

Low Carb, No Sugar, Low Fat

Whole grains, beans, fruits and vegetables are essential. Cut on food like pasta, bread, rice and alcohol. Moderate amounts of meat and nuts are fine to enjoy. No sugar! Be careful with fruits that are high in sugar. Best to eat berries (any kind), kiwi, cantaloupe which are low in sugar. Use stevia as your sugar substitute. It is important that you familiarize yourself with the food calorie tables, which can be easily obtained by searching the internet.

Wear tight clothing and wear a belt!
You will most likely stop eating more if you feel your clothes are tight! A reminder that you are overweight.

Eat 3 Healthy Meals on a set schedule daily
Eat BEFORE you are hungry!

DIET PROGRAM - STAGE I

Supplements

1. *The Thin Factors* – **(Leptin Resistance)**
   Too often, we overeat because the hypothalamus—the appetite center of the brain--is slow to receive those "stop right there!" signals. The hormone leptin acts like a biochemical traffic cop, helping regulate metabolism and energy intake. Like a cleaning crew, The Thin Factors essentially scrubs and tidies up the dirty leptin receptors, enabling them to work with brisk efficiency and fosters a sense of satisfaction to foil phony hunger pangs. **The hormonal signals reach the brain with greater speed, so metabolism, regulated by the hypothalamus, returns to healthy function.** *Two capsules a half an hour before you eat will almost alleviate any chance of over eating.*

2. *Max Metabolism* – **(Thyroid Resistance)**
   Helps to naturally re-establish normal metabolism and increases energy level. Resulting in **more burned up calories and faster weight loss.** It is your natural thermostat, a super energizer, it turbo-charges your metabolism to burn the fat you don't want. *One to two capsules 1 hour before each meal* super charges your metabolism, to kick start your fat burning potential.

3. *Craving Factor* – **(Adrenaline Resistance)**
   Is a unique combination of "**Washing Minerals**" and special "**Healing Vitamin Peptides**" to clean and rejuvenate your intestinal and colon to relieve constipation, food allergies, and healthy repair of your digestion, it even curbs cravings! *Dissolve 1 teaspoon in 16 ounces of water. On an empty stomach in the morning before breakfast and again in the evening before dinner. Drink **5 bottles per day** throughout the day maintain your hydration level is imperative.* Make sure you drink lots of water. **The more water you drink the more fat is flushed. That's it!** You're on your way to cleansing your system!

4. *The Slimming Fat Burn Cream* – **(Thyroid Resistance)**
   7-Keto - Scientifically Backed Active Ingredient
   - ➤ 300% more weight loss than diet and exercise alone
   - ➤ Majority of weight loss is fat loss
   - ➤ Promotes weight loss without use of stimulants
   - ➤ Active ingredient awarded a U.S. Patent for weight loss
   - ➤ Increase metabolism without the use of Stimulants

   Rub 3-4 pumps of Slimming Fat Burn Cream on areas needed help to lose inches, AM & PM

5. *Weight & Inches* – **(Insulin Resistance)**
   Helps to jump start metabolism using all natural green tea extract improves metabolic rate with Polyphenols and ECGC, which contain powerful antioxidant properties and help stimulate and improve your metabolism. Using Ginsenosides, a specific extraction that Normalizes the **internal "switch"** and allows the stomach to quickly respond when you eat, Weight & Inches helps regulate a dysfunctional system and virtually eliminates the possibility of overeating. *One capsule a half an hour before eating gives your stomach the extra push it needs.* Suddenly that extra piece of pie doesn't seem so inviting.

6. *Max Performance Specialist* – **(Insulin Resistance & Energy Balance)** Cordyceps radically increases cellular energy by 30%, the traditional Chinese doctors would use *Cordyceps* mushroom to **energize, improve health, and balance glucose level.** *Take 1or 2 tablets 3 times daily with food.*

7. *"Daily Energy"* & *"Daily Wellness"* – **(Vitamins & Minerals)** While you're dieting you may not be getting the recommended vitamins and minerals. That's why we suggest Daily Energy and Daily Wellness as part of your "Daily" routine. Packed full of vital vitamins and minerals. It will help your succeed in your day and your diet!!! Just take two tablets of "Daily Wellness" and two tablets of *"Daily Energy" twice a day and feel the difference.*

8. *Max Sea & Super B12* – **Supply extra Energy to Burn Extra Fat**
   Helps to increase energy while on a diet.

DIET PROGRAM - STAGE II

Congratulations!!!

**You've finished Stage I of our Weight Loss Program
for at least two months. You've watched yourself lose those
unwanted and unattractive inches and now you're ready for...**

DIET PROGRAM - STAGE II

The Hunger Factor **and the 500 calorie** a day Diet
Only for 40 Days!

Will change your body & your "satiety brain"

HUNGER FACTOR

**Special proprietary blend of natural ingredients
Formulated by Prof. Dr. Paul Ling Tai**

**1. To Re-Program the Satiety Center by cleansing
and re-starting your new eating habits.**

**2. Burns the bad white fat that produces
inflammation and washes them out of your body.**

500 CALORIE DIET
NO Sugar, No Fat, No Carb

It can be done! You're not going to starve...

Hunger Factor plus continuing all of the **supplements
of Stage I Diet** is going to change your whole perspective on
eating. Eating a 500 calorie nutritional diet will allow your body
to optimally use the stored fat. It's pretty simple. **Take out the
sugars, fats and carbs** in your everyday diet and your body will
have no choice but to use & Burn the "bad fat" for fuel, leaving you
only curves "in the right places".

**Ok...Ok...Sounds great...But 500 calories...
What can I eat?**

There are still many choices available on your road to success. Veggies, fruits and lean proteins are vital in maintain a healthy nutritionally complete body. One 3 ounce serving of lean beef, veal, chicken, or fresh white fish are great sources of protein giving you what you need to conquer the day!   Listed below are fruits and veggies that are great for your body and low in calories. Each fruit or veggie and or lean protein is considered 1 item.   Don't forget you're allowed to have up to 8 items a day. But 2 servings of fruits or 2 servings of proteins may not be eaten together at the same time. 2 vegetables together are ok.

FRUITS
Please remember you need to follow the suggest serving

1 apple or a handful of strawberries or a ½ grapefruit or 1 Fresh peach or a ½ cup of dried apricots or 2 plums

VEGETABLES
Please remember you need to follow the suggested serving

Broccoli, Celery, fennel, Cabbage, Cucumbers, Green/red peppers, Spinach, Green Beans, Cauliflower, ½ cup radishes, Onions/garlic, Lettuce, Asparagus, ½ cup eggplant, ½ of a tomato

The following crackers are allowed but remember – You may only choose one item per meal!

1 Ryvita Crispbread or 4 stone ground wheat thins or 1 Melba toast or 1 Kavali crispbread or soda crackers

"I've eaten so many fruits and veggies I think I'm becoming a rabbit!!

You can substitute ¾ of a cup of unflavored non-fat yogurt in place of one of your fruits or vegetables. If you desire you may sweeten with our Health Secrets Sweet Therapy, there is not suggested amount of sweet therapy, you may use to your discretion.   You may also use 3 eggs (1 whole plus 2 whites) or ½ cup of fat- free cottage cheese as your protein occasionally! No more than once daily!

NO oil, NO butter, NO gravy NO dressing of any kind may be used. You may use the juice of a lemon or lime with each meal if desired along with apple cider vinegar with sweetener substitute. There are many spices and herbs that can be used in place. They are better for you and all natural. Most are ok but here is a few of our favorites - *Salt/pepper, Mustard powder, Sweet basil, Parsley, Thyme, marjoram.*

Please remember that while you're on *Stage II* of your weight loss plan you still need to remain taking your *Stage I* Supplements. *Stage II* only lasts for 40 days. After that, you will have a new lease on life and a better understanding of what your body truly needs to stay lean and healthy.

DIET PROGRAM - STAGE II- 40 DAYS

Supplements

1. *Hunger Factor* – Take one dose by mouth in early morning & one dose in PM daily on empty stomach

2. *The Thin Factors* - Two capsules a half an hour before you eat

3. *Max Metabolism* – One to two capsules half an hour before each meal

4. *Craving Factor* – Dissolve 1 level teaspoon in 8 ounces of water. You must drink 5 16oz bottles of water daily to wash away your fat (2 in the morning, 2 in the afternoon, and 1 at night)

5. *Max Sea* - 15 drops with water twice daily

6. *Super B12* - 3 sprays AM & Noon

7. *Daily Energy & Daily Wellness* - **Two tablets of each, twice a day**

8. *Max Performance:* 1 tablet 3 times daily

Day 1 and 2 - Take HCG/Hunger Factor and eat well
Starting with **Day 3:**

Take HCG/Hunger Factor and follow **500 calorie for up to 40 days** (except during menstruation: do not take HCG/Hunger Factor, but do continue the 500 calorie diet)

You must stay on this diet for **no less than 30 days**. If you only need to lose 5 pounds, you may use **Stage I only** to achieve the result, but you must stay on it for 30 days even if you already reached your goal in 3 weeks. It seems that even in the mildest cases of obesity the Satiety center requires about 30 days to reset the eating pattern which has been previously set in order to regain fully its normal eating pattern. Please keep these 30 days, no cheating, consecutive, effective HCG/Hunger Factor days of 500 calorie diet in mind if you want to affect your metabolism both during the protocol and for the rest of your life.

Set Your Weight Point!

Besides seriously avoiding sugars and starches during the three weeks following the HCG/Hunger Factor Stage II phase, even if you don't go over your maintenance weight, you should attempt to keep your weight as steady as possible during this phase to reach a new **Set Weight Point** in your body. It seems the faster this is done and the more consistent one stays at a weight, the quicker the body sets and maintains the new weight. This is when we want our bodies to take on the new **Set Weight Point**.

Avoiding sugars and starches also helps us achieve the goal of maintaining weight loss because most people crave less and are satisfied with less than when they chose to indulge.

HCG INJECTIONS vs. SUBLINGUAL (under the tongue)

Until recently, most participants found injections to be the only consistent, effective method of using HCG/Hunger Factor for weight loss. However, support of **sublingual HCG/Hunger Factor is becoming more popular** and getting better reviews among HCG/ Hunger Factor dieters. The method of mixing and supplies are slightly different for the different methods. So, you must decide which method you are going to use before ordering and mixing your HCG/Hunger Factor.

Adjustment to HCG/Hunger Factor dosage during a cycle
Sublingual dosage is generally 125 i.u. twice daily.
Many participants increase the daily dosage strength by taking a
125 i.u. dosage 3 times daily (waiting a day or two in between
adjustments) for one or more of the following reasons:

- The participant continues to be very hungry after the first week when hunger should be less
- Energy continues to be quite low (May need to increase Max Metabolism and Super B12).
- Slow weight loss
- Slight signs of immunity
- Potency - Hunger Factor's potency last longer if stay in the refrigerator.

Proper HCG/Hunger Factor Storage
Prior to mixing, the HCG/Hunger Factor should be kept in a
dark box at refrigerator temperature until expiration date. Several
companies report expiration dates about three years from current
date. **Once HCG/Hunger Factor has been mixed, it must be
stored in the refrigerator and should be potent for at least 30
days** although some brands will claim longer potency.

*Warning: While some participants in the past have
been advised to freeze HCG until you are ready
to use it, this is generally not accepted as proper
storage and may affect potency. DO NOT FREEZE
HCG.*

STAGE II DIET SUGGESTIONS

Breakfast: Tea or coffee in any quantity without sugar. A non-caloric sweetener or Stevia may be used.

Lunch: 1. 100 grams/3oz. of veal, beef, chicken breast, fresh white fish, lobster, crab or shrimp. All visible fat must be carefully removed before cooking, and the meat must be weighed raw. It must be broiled or grilled without additional fat.

2. Chose of the following Vegetables: spinach, chard, chicory, beet greens, green salad, tomatoes, celery, fennel, onions, red radishes, cucumbers, asparagus, cabbage, salads and beans.

3. One breadstick (grissini) or one Melba toast.

4. An apple or handful of strawberries or one half grapefruit, 1/2 orange

Dinner: The same four choices as lunch can be used for dinner.

The juice of one lemon daily is allowed for all purposed. Salt, pepper, vinegar, mustard, garlic, sweet basil, parsley, thyme, marjoram, etc., may be used for seasoning, but no oil, butter or dressing. Check ingredients for hidden sugar and oils.

Unsweetened tea, coffee, plain water, or mineral water are the only drinks allowed, but they may be taken in any quantity and at all times.

DO NOT FORGET - You should **drink minimum 2 liters/ quarts of these fluids per day in (5) divided 16oz/500ml bottles.** Many patients are afraid to drink so much because they fear that this may make them retain more water. This is a wrong notion as the body is more inclined to store water when the intake falls below its normal requirements.

The fruit or the breadstick may be eaten between meals instead of with lunch or dinner, but not more than four items listed for lunch and dinner may be eaten at one meal.

There is no objection to breaking up the two meals. For instance having a breadstick and an apple for breakfast or before going to bed, provided they are deducted from the regular meals. The whole daily ration of two breadsticks or two fruits may not be eaten at the same time, nor can any item saved from the previous day be added on the following day. In the beginning, patients are advised to check every meal against their diet sheet before starting to eat and not to rely on their memory. **Keep a diary of the food eaten.** It is also worth

pointing out that any attempt to observe this diet without HCG/
Hunger Factor will lead to trouble in two to three days.

**No restriction on the size of one apple. Maximum 2 apples
a day, at least 4 hours apart.**

Making up the 1200 Calories for Stage I or 500 calories for Stage II

The diet used in **Stage I** must not exceed 1200 calories per
day. For **Stage II**, do not exceed 500 calories per day. For instance,
if a patient drops the apple and eats extra breadstick instead, he will
not be getting more calories but he will not lose weight. **Do not
exchange carbohydrate and sugar content of foods you eat in
the diet.**

150 grams portion size of protein for Stage I & 100 grams or 3.5 oz portion of Protein for Stage II

In America, lean cut of beef, i.e. flank steak, tenderloin, low-
grade veal should be used for one meal, and fish, chicken breast,
lobster, crawfish, prawns or shrimp, or crabmeat for the other
meal. Where the Italian breadsticks, the so called grissini, are not
available, one Melba toast may be used instead; through they are
psychologically less satisfying. A Melba toast has about the same
weight as the very porous grissini which is much more to look at and
to chew.

When local conditions or the feeding habits of the population
make changes necessary it must be borne in mind that the total daily
intake must not exceed 1200 calories for Stage I and 500 calories
for Stage II. If the best possible results are to be obtained, the daily
ration should contain no more than 150 grams of fat-free protein and
a minimal amount of starch for Stage I and 100 grams of protein per
meal for Stage II.

Just as the daily dose of HCG/Hunger Factor is the same in
all cases, so the same diet proves to be satisfactory for a woman of
smaller stature or a tough working muscular man. **Under the effect
of HCG/Hunger Factor the obese body is always able to obtain
all the calories it needs from the abnormal fat deposits.**
Because we are burning those extra fat we have been storing on
our waist, thighs, butt, etc. they must all be burned off for a new
"sculpted body".

Feel good with the right food

The most popular foods in American culture are pizza, white bread, sugary foods, cookies, sodas, cakes and all other foods high on the glycemic index. They are also foods that cause blood sugar levels to rise quickly, and subsequently fall quickly. More sugar results in more carbohydrate cravings. The more chocolate you eat, the more you will want to eat. By avoiding sugary carbohydrates altogether, you can lower stress levels, lose weight and control the cortisol produced by your adrenal glands.

Fried foods

Compelling you to doze off instead of accomplishing your goals for the day, oily foods can induce a tired, deadbeat feeling. People who have depended on fried and greasy foods for most of their lives can expect a heavier load of cleanup work than those who watched what they ate. By eating balanced meals packed with vitamins and minerals you will feel like a cleaner, lighter person.

Eating foods high in sugar, starch and grease you are risking a lifetime of good health for a few minutes of taste bud satisfaction. Excess high glycemic carbohydrates and transfats are allergic, inflammatory and diabetes inducers, Stay Away from these food!

Severe food restriction

As observed within the Stage II HCG/Hunger Factor protocol, enhances fat burning from stomach and lower limbs, improving the obtained results. These major short term changes (500 calorie diet) yield long term results (extra weight gone) and very little carryover baggage (Individuals could expect to eat when they were hungry and not regain the weight back). **Bravo!**

As you enter the **maintenance phase**, you eat as you wish with the exception of no sugars and no starches (carbohydrates are acceptable), but you weigh yourself everyday to make sure you haven't gained more than 2 pounds since your last HCG date weight. Pretty simple!

In time (about 2 months) you can add slowly low glycemic carbohydrates gradually without gaining weight because your metabolism reached equilibrium to your **SET WEIGHT**.

The final step is to slowly add sugars and starches. As before, you must weigh everyday to make sure you haven't gained more than 2 pounds since your last Stage II weight.

Enjoy your New Body!

Real Success Stories..

Dr. Maria S.
Total Lost: 25 lbs.
Best Feature: New sculpted Body Shape!

38 years old, a doctor and athlete, unable to lose weight on stomach, butt, and thighs, was unhappy with her inability to lose weight in spite of dieting and daily exercise. **On Stage I**, she lost **7 pounds** in **30 DAYS!** Unbelievable result!

On Stage II, she lost **18 pounds** in **40 DAYS!** But most importantly, she saw an extraordinary loss of inches around her stomach, butt, and thighs, and for the first time, she has the body shape that she wanted! It is not just the weight but lost a lot of inches. Another successful story!

Cathie's Weight Loss Data

Cathie's experience with Stage I

Starting weight: 165lbs
Ending weight: 136 lbs *(Total- Lost 34 lbs in 2 month period)*
Dress size: went from *large size 12* to a *small size 8*

46 years old female Dental Assistant, gained a lot of weight after the birth of her 2nd child. Unable to lose the weight in spite of many diets. Her problems were mostly fat on her arms, stomach and shoulders. She went on Stage I with the 1200 calories diet, she lost **7 pounds** in **30 DAYS!** A happy ending!

Best meals:
  a. Breakfast: coffee with fat free *Coffemate*, Berries
  b. Lunch: V8 juice, 3oz ham/chicken breast, or turkey breast lunchmeat, *Wasa* bread, coffee w/ fat free *Coffemate and salads*
  c. Supper: 3oz grilled chicken breast, steamed broccoli & salads
  d. Snack: diet *Jell-O, sugar and fat free*
Cut out Diet Soda from diet- switched to tea

Supplements taken:
AM (Hunger Factor Liquid) Sublingual
  a. Craving Factor - 1 tsp in a 16oz bottle of water or tea
  b. (2) Max Metabolism–capsules
  c. (2) The Thin Factors –gel caps
  d. (1) Daily Energy –tablets
  e. (1) Daily Wellness – tablets
One hour before lunch
  a) Craving Factor - 1 tsp in a 16oz bottle of water or tea
  b) (2) Max Metabolism – capsules
  c) (2) The Thin Factors –gel caps
  d) (1) Daily Energy – tablets
  e) (1) Daily Wellness – tablets
  Mid-afternoon - Craving Factor - 1 tsp in a 16oz bottle of water or tea

One hour before supper (Hunger Factor Liquid) Sublingual
    a) Craving Factor - 1 tsp in a 16oz bottle of water or tea
    b) (2) The Thin Factors – gel caps
    c) (2) Max Metabolism – capsules

Tips from Cathie's Success:
*Buddy up with someone, they are supportive and more fun.
*Don't skip meals! By eating every meal your body's
metabolism stay rev up and burning.
*Drink lots of water with Craving Factor - Body needs a minimum
of 2-3 quarts of water per day to survive.
*Take "Before" pictures and measurements, you will see results -
Yes! You can't remember exactly the way it was - "Before" pictures
are Good Reminders!
*Daily Energy and Daily Wellness really helped to keep energy
level up! Use Super B12, 3-4 sprays AM & Noon or whenever
feel tired - Energy is absolutely necessary to burn the fat you don't
need.
*Be sure to measure out your portions or you'll over eat. You will
be surprised that a small amount can be filling!
* Keep a diary of what you eat and how much you eat! You
will be surprised of the amount of food you forget you ate!

Cathie's Personal Comments:

*Cathie
After Losing 34
pounds! What A
Super Body!*

*I was never a water drinker before.
But now, I crave water!
I used to drink 5-6 cans of diet
mountain dew a day, don't even
want it now.*

*Love seeing the pounds off 1-2
lbs at a time! Getting off those
pounds is a lot of fun when you can
actually see the pounds drop off!*

*Be careful trying to go back eating
a lot of Carbs and sugar. They
made me want to eat more.*

Beckie B. (R.N.)'s Happy Ending!

Total - Lost 30 lbs. (14kg) - WOW! Did you say 30lbs??
Lost 21 inches (53cm)
From a Size 18-20 to a Size 14-16

Cursed? She tried every diet on earth - could not lose weight!!!

START DATE: 4/12/2009	211 lbs/96kg
END DATE: 08/11/2009	181 lbs/82kg
TOTAL WEIGHT LOSS:	30 Lbs/14kg

INCHES LOSS:
    Bust lost 5"/12.7cm
    Waist lost 3.5"/8.89cm
    Hips lost 5"/12.7cm	

4/12/2009	**8/11/2009**
BUST- 47"/119cm	BUST-42"/107cm = Lost 5"/12.7cm
WAIST- 37"/94cm	WAIST-40.5"/103cm = Lost 3.5"/8.89cm
HIPS- 50"/127cm	HIPS-45"/114cm = Lost 5"/13cm
RIGHT THIGH- 28.5"/72cm	RIGHT THIGH-26"/66cm = Lost 2.5"/6cm
LEFT THIGH- 29"/74cm	LEFT THIGH-26"/66cm = Lost 3"/8cm
RIGHT ARM-13.5"/34.30cm	RIGHT ARM- 12.5"/31.75cm = Lost 1"/2.54cm
LEFT ARM- 13.5"/34.30cm	LEFT ARM- 12.5"/31.75cm = Lost 1"/2.54cm

Mrs. Ivani O. - She was Desperate to Lose Weight!!!

58 years old, Menopause. Desperate and Angry!!! She has been to 4 different Weight Loss doctors, all unsuccessful. Big problem with her stomach, waistline and thighs and arms.
On Stage I - She lost 8 lbs - Excellent Result!
On Stage II - she lost *39 pounds* in **50 DAYS!!!**

*Total **47** pounds!* Job well done! Congratulations! Mrs. Ivani worked hard to stay on the exercise program and adjusted to higher dose of Max Metabolism and Super B12 3 times a day when feeling tired. It's now 6 months after and she is still the same weight! By the way, she found a new boyfriend who is crazy about her!

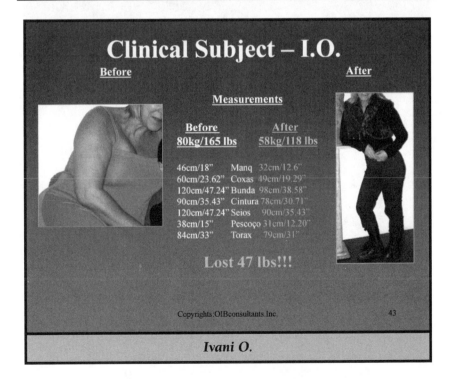

Clinical Subject – I.O.

Before

After

Measurements

Before		After
80kg/165 lbs		**58kg/118 lbs**
46cm/18"	Manq	32cm/12.6"
60cm/23.62"	Coxas	49cm/19.29"
120cm/47.24"	Bunda	98cm/38.58"
90cm/35.43"	Cintura	78cm/30.71"
120cm/47.24"	Seios	90cm/35.43"
38cm/15"	Pescoço	31cm/12.20"
84cm/33"	Torax	79cm/31"

Lost 47 lbs!!!

43

Ivani O.

Dr. L.S. - Amazing Staying Power!

On Stage I
37 years old Dentist, mother of a cute daughter,
overweight most of her life, unsuccessful in controlling her diet.
She lost **8 pounds** on **Stage I** in **30 DAYS!** Horray!

On Stage II
she lost **27 pounds** in **40 DAYS!!!** Just incredible!

Total - Lost 35 pounds & Lots of inches in 70 Day!
She made it to her Dental School re-union with a new
practice, new body, and maybe to some colleagues, a
new person!

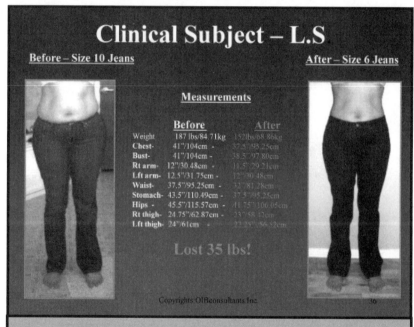

Clinical Subject – L.S

Before – Size 10 Jeans   **After – Size 6 Jeans**

Measurements

	Before	After
Weight	187 lbs/84.71kg	152lbs/68.86kg
Chest-	41"/104cm -	37.5"/95.25cm
Bust-	41"/104cm -	38.5"/97.80cm
Rt arm-	12"/30.48cm -	11.5"/29.21cm
Lft arm-	12.5"/31.75cm -	12"/30.48cm
Waist-	37.5"/95.25cm -	32"/81.28cm
Stomach-	43.5"/110.49cm -	37.5"/95.25cm
Hips -	45.5"/115.57cm -	41.75"/106.05cm
Rt thigh-	24.75"/62.87cm -	23"/58.42cm
Lft thigh-	24"/61cm -	22.25"/56.52cm

Lost 35 lbs!

Copyrights:OIBconsultants Inc.

36

Dr. L.S.
2 Months Later, A Follow Up with L.S. - She stayed on the
maintenance program and was thrilled that she was able to
retain the weight loss! She did not gain any weight!

SHOPPING LIST FOR STAGE I & II DIETS

Splenda or Stevia
Montreal steak seasoning
Montreal chicken seasoning
Italian spices
White wine vinegar
Red wine vinegar
Heinz Spicy brown mustard
Red hot sauce
Soy sauce (Kikoman)
Lemon juice
Minced garlic
Celery seed

Beef bouillon cubes
Chicken bouillon cubes
Cup a soup
Murrays sugar free chocolate
cookie packs- 70 cal
SF Jello - Sugar free
SF Jello pudding - Sugar free
SF popsicles - Sugar free
SF Edy's juice bars - Sugar free
Fruit leather

Crystal light (any flavor) -
  Sugar free
V8 juice
Fat free half and half
Iced coffee

Apples (braeburn are great!)
Cantaloupe
Strawberries
Nectarines
Plums
Blueberries, any berry

Wasa light crackers
Melba toast (all flavors)
Grissini sticks (Italian)

Frozen broccoli steamers
Frozen broccoli and
cauliflower steamers
Coleslaw - No sugar
Broccoli slaw
Celery
 Cucumbers
Red, yellow, orange, and green
bell peppers
Fresh baby spinach
Onions
Green beans
Canned Rotelle tomatoes with
green chilies or fire roasted
tomatoes
Rotisserie chicken - remove
skin and fat
Turkey/chicken lunchmeat
Sirloin burger
Flank steak
Chicken breast - skinless
Boneless pork chops -
  cut out fat
Frozen Tilapia
Ham steaks
Egg beaters
Fat free cottage cheese
Yogurts - Sugar free
  and low fat

RECIPES FOR STAGE 2 DIET

Marinated Flank steak
In large (1 gal) ziplock bag, mix: ¼ c soy sauce, 2 Tbsp. white vinegar, 1 tsp. Splenda, 1 heaping Tbsp. minced garlic, and 10 drops of Red hot sauce.
Coat both sides of flank steak generously with Montreal Steak seasoning.
Place flank steak into bag with marinade.
Marinate for 24 hours, and then grill.
Serve sliced very thin against the grain.

Marinated Chicken
In large (1 gal) ziplock bag, mix: Heinz spicy brown mustard, 2 Tbsp. white vinegar, 1 tsp. Splenda, 1 Tbsp. water.
Coat chicken breast with Montreal Chicken seasoning.
Place chicken breast into bag with marinade.
Marinate for 24 hours, and then grill chicken along with large slices of onion.
Serve with slices of grilled onion.

Spicy Tilapia with Spinach and Tomatoes
Cook Tilapia until almost cooked.
In Sautee pan combine: 1 Tbsp. minced garlic, and 2 cans of Rotelle tomatoes with green chilies (or substitute fire roasted tomatoes for less spice).
Sautee until hot.
In Sautee pan: place Tilapia on top of tomato mixture and mound with fresh spinach.
Cover and cook until fish is cooked/flaky.
Serve.

SALAD DRESSINGS
WINNERS WITHOUT OIL & SUGAR

Coleslaw Dressing
½ cup White vinegar
¼ cup water
3-4 Tbsp. Splenda
Celery seed
Black pepper

Red wine Dressing
¾ cup red wine vinegar
1 Tbsp. minced garlic
Italian spices
2 Tbsp. Splenda

Mustard Dressing
4 Tablespoons Vinegar of Choice
2 Tablespoons Yellow Mustard
1 Packet of Splenda or Stevia
¼ tsp. of salt
(Author's favorite)

Katherine Lee - From Fat to Trim...

I am very excited to tell you that I lost 25 pounds!!! But even more important, I lost a lot of inches, all in the right places!

I went from a very tight size 10 to a size 6!!! A waitress called me TINY!!! Can you believe it!

That's right! I did it! and I am proud of myself. 9 months later, I have not gained 1 lb. back! That's totally never happened to me before!

Ok, stop here for a moment.... I can see your skeptical look now. You probably are thinking that I am just another one of those incredible stories just to get you to buy some weight loss products... and that it is not going to happen for you.

Well, maybe you are right that this diet is not for you... It is not for you because you are not committed to lose weight, but if you are serious, this diet can help you.

Please allow me to share my story with you...

I was not obese. I was not extremely fat. But I was a very tight size 10 who refused to buy the next bigger size... somehow, I thought I could just squeeze all the flabby body parts into my size 10 pants and zipped it up... Ouch! My zipper caught the excess flesh!!! That's it!!! Where is that pair of scissor!

I, like many of you, can gain weight just by breathing air! And being a menopausal 57 years old women, it is like adding oil to the fire... you can exercise and diet all you want, but those fat seems to cling onto my body like honey to bees.

I started to Dream about what I'll look like when I reach my weight-loss goal. I also spent more time reading fashion magazines; Vogue, Elle, InStyle, Barzar... Those skinny models and movie stars were my goal! They were my inspiration, my stimulation, and my obsession! **You've got to be obsessed with the idea that you are going to lose weight, otherwise, you will fail.**

Through Prof. Dr. Tai's extensive research he developed natural formulas to help solve weight loss and obesity from the root. He has **a scientific approach to weight loss.**

According to Prof. Dr. Tai, to know how to lose the fat in your body, we first must first study to understand all about Fat. He did. Dr. Tai uncovered the **4 Resistance Factors** to weight loss and obesity.

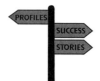

Katherine M. Lee
"My Personal Journey – From Fat to Trim"

*"**Weight**" has always been a problem word for me... ever since I was a little girl; I was the "Fat" one in the family. My older sister was beautiful, fit and trim; my younger sister was not born yet and my younger brother was never able to gain weight no matter how much my mom fed him! But me, **I loved to eat**... I ate alongside my brother, and finished what he didn't. Sometimes I ate till I was rolling on the floor in pain, But then I seemed to have forgotten all about the unbearable pain and start eating again!*

*Why did I love food so much??? I used to hate people calling me "**Fat girl**". I didn't want anyone to talk about my "Weight". I want them to leave me alone and just let me eat!*

When I turned 13, like all the teenager girls in the world, I discovered "boys"! I started to spend more time looking at myself in the mirror, and my mirror was not very kind to me... I kept seeing this pudgy body of mine and that image is still haunting till today!!! I started to worry about not having any one want to date me. "Who's going to ask a fat girl out???" Believe me, there were lots of pressure growing up in Hong Kong, with those skinny Asian girls; compared to them, I was fat!

But I loved food - A LOT of food! And since I work so hard every day, I felt that I deserved to have my favorite foods as a reward for all my hard work. I prayed to God for the privilege to eat all I wanted without gaining any weight. But I guess God knew better, he didn't allow me to eat without showing me the other side of my behavior... my scale dipping drastically to the right!

Well, that's when my diet journey started and it was **a never ending vicious cycle of daily starvation, exercise, and deprivation of food** till I couldn't bear it, and then I told myself, "I'm just going to have a small little bite, which lead to a bigger bite; pretty soon, the whole cake was gone. I had to finish the whole cake or I feel guilty leaving something behind.

I was always "pudgy" but I never thought that I was "overweight". I was able to maintain a size 10 body; sometimes very tight size 10 –I warned my family to watch themselves for flying buttons! Other times my size 10 clothes fitted me just right, I don't need to lose weight! I was proud and happy to be a size 10 at age 57!

So what made me decide to lose some weight?
It was a challenge by Prof. Dr. Tai, the perfectionist who always striving for excellence and always searching for the best secret ingredients. He has helped doctors and their patients all over the world with his special natural supplements. He is called "the Doctor's Doctor".

Through his research and studies, he found that there

is not a single culprit to weight gain; therefore, a single diet pill just doesn't work. I'm sure you and I have a drawer full of diet pills to prove it!

Prof. Dr. Tai's 2 Stage Diet Program targets the **4 different "Resistance" that our body creates.** I found his theory interesting, and made a lot of sense, so I decided to give it a go. Why? Because if it works for me, it will work for anyone! **I have tried for almost 50 years to lose those 10 extra pounds and failed every time.** I finally settled decided to be happy with the size I was. So it would be very motivating to see if I can actually break that barrier.

Commitment, that's the key word to success! If you are not serious about losing weight, and following our diet program, don't bother getting started. **But if you're ready to finally look and feel the way you know you deserve to and you have at least 10 extra pounds to lose, then this is it for you!**

In the beginning it was tough, I was happy to have lost 10 pounds with the Stage I Diet program, but it took me 2 months. I didn't see any weight loss for almost 2 weeks, I was disappointed... a couple of days later, all of a sudden, my scale tipped several lines to the left!!! I couldn't believe my eyes!!! I was ecstatic!!! I was actually losing the weight!

Although I reached my goal of losing 10 pounds, but **I wanted to see what it would be like to be "skinny"** – a word I never have associated it with myself. I was excited to start the Stage II diet program!

My excitement quickly diminished when I saw that **I was only allowed 500 calories a day while on Stage II?!** One candy bar would be 500 calories and it only lasted me 3 minutes!!! There is no way that I can stay on a 500 calorie diet!!!" I'll starve to death!!! I was annoyed with such a requirement!!! It's just impossible!

Prof. Dr. Tai smiled and said: "But you only have to do Stage II for 40 days! **Can you just give up 40 days of eating pleasure to achieve your lifetime dream?"**

That did it! 40 days wasn't too much of a challenge... **I've been on some kind of a diet my whole life. And most of them have lasted months what's another 40 days?**

Prof. Dr. Tai's "Hunger Factor" is the key to the Stage II diet program. I lost 15 pounds in 1 month!!! **Not only did I lose a total of 25 pounds, I lost it in the right places...** Suddenly those little annoying bulges of fat on my upper back were gone. My arms didn't keep waving long after I had stopped! My hips, my thighs and most importantly my waist! **I have never had a 28 inch waist** before and at 57!!! I was so proud of myself I felt good, healthy and most importantly, I achieved my goal.

How did I stay on a 500 calories daily diet? Well, I played a game with myself. I pretended that the 500 calories a day were dollars and every day, I have to budget myself on how to spend them. Do I really want that pizza, for 310 calories a slice? It would be great right now But later I'd be starving. OR, I could have one cup of Lipton package Chicken noodle soup at 45 calories, 3 pieces of Melba toast at 60 calories, 1 medium red apple at 95 calories, 6 slices (5gram) of packaged low calorie shaved ham for 45 calories, and two teaspoons of mustard with 10 calories, all that for only 255 calories!!! I decided with my brain and not my stomach and opted for the second. I was full and happy.

I was encouraged to continue when I saw my weight and inches slipping right away!!! I'm excited to wake up in the morning. I can't wait to go and see my new friend, **my scale**, The progress in front of me is amazing!!

And my clothes...can you believe this. My tailor is tired of seeing me... all of my dresses, pants, and suits have been taken in 3 times!!! It was such a thrill seeing myself in the mirror; people kept telling me how skinny I am!!! It was unbelievable! Wait...ME?! **At the age of 57, most people are overweight and saggy, but I'm getting the looks and complements.**

I looked at my older pictures, I was shocked! I can't believe my eyes what I was thinking? How did I let myself get that out of control? What was wrong with my head? I am embarrassed to show my fat picture.... **Oh, those double chins, and rolls, gosh! It was awful!**

I'm on a maintenance program now. I still take all the Stage I supplements but at a lower dosage; I eat about 1200 to 1500 calories a day and I've learned **it's not necessarily what you eat just how much.**

My body and mind are now trained to look at food with a more critical eye and I've learned to be more careful with my food choices. It has been 9 months since I finished my Stage II Diet Program, and I am delighted to report to you that I haven't gain my weight back!

A thousand dollars may give me happiness for a day or two, but shedding those extra 25pounds worth more than a thousand dollars to me. It is by far the biggest thrill I have ever had in my life! I am now a proud and happy size 6!

Thank you Prof. Dr. Tai! You made my dream come true!

Katherine M. Lee

President
Health Secrets USA
November, 2009

I Lost 25 lbs!!!

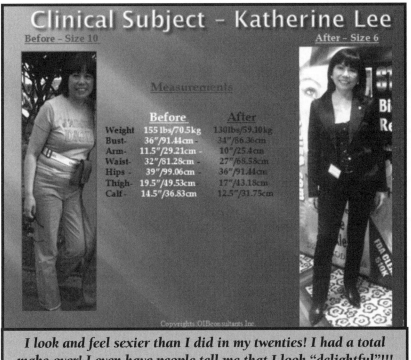

I look and feel sexier than I did in my twenties! I had a total make-over! I even have people tell me that I look "delightful"!!!

Waist lost - 5"
Hips lost - 3"

Chapter Twenty-Three

UNDERSTANDING HOW TO EAT FOR OPTIMAL RESULTS

Burning The Fat

To be fit and lose fat, understand this one extremely important point: ***To lose inches and weight, you must burn fat. To burn fat, your body must burn sugar first. Your body won't burn any fat until it has finished burning sugar first.***

That's right, the secret to burning fat is knowing the sequence the body goes through to burn off the excess calories. Now, you'll know when and how to eat for your maximum fitness ratio.

1. The body burns the stored sugar from the muscles.
2. Then it moves to burning the excess sugar stored in the liver.
3. Only after those sugars are gone will the body start burning the visceral fat inside the body.

To make this conversion happen for the best results, follow these dietary guidelines that I'll expand in the following chapters.

You must eat if you feel hungry. If you don't, your body thinks you are starving and shifts down your metabolic rate, just like you shift gears downward from third to decelerate to first when your car comes to a stop. Good for the car, but bad for your body, because this makes everything worse as you won't burn any calories.

• **Seek a four-hour block of time to not eat** large amounts of food and allow this free-eating zone for digestion and fat burning.

• **When you feel hungry, first drink** 16 ounces of water or iced tea. Better yet, drink the water with a heaping teaspoon of **Craving Factor** and wait ten minutes.

- **Go ahead** with a salad with an olive oil and lemon-based dressing with spices if you are still hungry after the iced tea? This will help with hunger, but it won't add too much sugar to your muscles and liver.

- **A protein-based diet** is a very IMPORTANT because it satisfies hunger and it kicks up metabolism.

- **THE THIN FACTORS must be used** to clean away the satiety center for hunger cravings; otherwise you will be munching all the time.

Burning fat is the heart of any weight loss. If we can't learn to do this, we will NEVER succeed!

Center Stage - Metabolism

Let's go deeper into what happens in your metabolism after you eat a meal and then apply what we know to your healthy eating habits.

Scene One – Digestion is first scene, and the hypothalamus receives signals from your body about whether you're hungry or not, so that your body can use energy to power itself. After you eat, the body first uses the glucose it needs immediately, and stores the rest. The body's glycogen from food and insulin is the pool for energy, and is stored in the liver and muscles.

If your blood glucose level falls, your pancreas stops releasing insulin, and then releases another G substance, glucagon, which converts the stored energy (glycogen) to sugar (glucose). So the effect is…when your intestinal gas tank empties of sugar, your body still supplies crucial energy to your central nervous system by converting glycogen to glucose.

Scene Two – The Fasting Phase, scene 2, is when you're sleeping or go long periods (over 4 hours) without eating. Your body is always in need for fuel and only stores about 300 calories in the *short-term* glycogen reservoir. Once you use up all of your available glucose during the digestive phase of metabolism, the body pulls from the longer-term storage in fatty tissue in the form of triglycerides (molecules that include a carbohydrate-containing glycerol). This keeps you going until you break the fast with breakfast. This is the important part to lose weight during overnight (over 8 hours of no food and unsweetened drinks).

Feasting allows our livers to store excess sugar as glycogen, so we can access energy without eating for hours. Once glycogen stores are full, we save the excess energy as fat. To break down fat, we first have to burn the glycogen, which can take a half hour of exercise, or not eating at all for 4 hours or more, and not drinking anything sweet. I always highly recommend water and unsweetened tea.

Scene Three - Slow the metabolic process, especially before your meal by having a little of the right kind of fats. When you get the hungry signals from the growling gut, you need to eat. However, that little growl doesn't tell you how much you should eat. You can slow down the appetite about twenty minutes before you eat by tricking your hormonal system. Do this by eating one of the three choices below and send the signal to your brain that you're full.

2 tabs of Omega-3
70 calories of fat in the form of six walnuts
Or twelve almonds
(Not during Stage II diet)

You'll stimulate production of CCK, which communicates with your brain and slows your stomach from emptying to keep you feeling full. CCK release and ghrelin reduction take about twenty minutes to kick in and take about 65 calories of fat to stimulate.

That way, you'll be able to sit down for a meal and eat for pleasure, not for hunger, which is one way to ensure you'll eat less. The average person is finished eating well before his satiety signals kick in, thus countering any possibility that his hormones can help him.

☞ *For the same reason, you should eat slowly. Chew and savor your food. Put your fork down, chew food slowly and thoroughly, and have a pleasant conversation with a friend or family. If you gulp down your food faster, you won't allow your satiety hormones time to kick in.*

Scene Four – Fiber, the last player on the metabolic stage, slows down the transit time of food and keeps you feeling full for a longer time. Ingesting 30 grams of fiber at breakfast helps you stay full until later afternoon. Great sources of fiber for breakfast are oatmeal, cereal, whole grains and non-sweet fruits, the vegetable or mushroom in an egg white omelet or a slice of whole grain bread.

Fiber controls blood sugar levels, lowers insulin levels, and lowers calorie intake for up to 18 hours a day. One study showed that you could lose nearly 6 lbs. in 8 weeks if you eat 1 gram of fiber an hour before each meal. Fiber and bulk from grains, seeds, and non-sweet fruits clear and detoxify the bowels. In the same sense, purified water serves your entire body to detoxify, hydrate, lubricate, and much more.

DOCTOR TAI'S IMPORTANT TIP

Flaxseeds can be used as a daily fiber supplement for bowel movements.

Buy small amounts, keep them refrigerated, and consume fresh as they tend to turn rancid if they sit too long. Flaxseed is an excellent source of oleic and linoleic acids, the essential fatty acids used widely to decrease inflammation. Take flax seeds in three ways:

Add them to your morning fruit smoothie or cereal.

Soak a teaspoon of seeds overnight and drink the brew,

water and seeds in the morning before eating.

In the evening, relax and unwind with a soothing cup of flax seed tea. First grind ¼ to ½ teaspoon of seeds (amount depends upon your taste buds) just like you would grind coffee beans. Pour the powder in a cup followed

hot water. Stir well and enjoy!

Chapter Twenty-Four
WEIGHT LOSS FOOD FACTS

Weight loss is more than just looking better. It's about being healthier, feeling stronger, and living longer
Dr. Tai

How Much Do You Know About Food?

Few of us are trained specifically in making good food choices or knowing instinctively what food is healthy for us. Many Americans confuse a portion of grain (like a helping of brown rice) for a breakfast cereal doused with sugar and milk for getting started every morning. The *Globesity* crisis is forcing us to wake up and take back our health by taking charge of our lives.

> ### The The Thin Factors Study – Case Three
> *Case 3, Jo, is a 59-year-old woman who lost 13 pounds, whittled her waistline from 43 to 37.5 inches, a net of -5.5 inches; and she lost an additional inch in her hip circumference. Her waist to hip ratio went from .915 to .815. The whole program in 90 days.* **Congratulations Jo !!!**

More and more, I am thrilled to see people willing to learn about nutrition and choosing freely to eat for themselves and not for their family, culture or because of their social circles. Eating for health and weight loss addiction is much like the sober, recovered alcoholic who must say, "no." Let's get food sober and recover from fat addictions. My intention here is to empower you as a well-informed consumer who can plan a healthy meal to maintain weight loss and prevent distress and disease.

Science of Nutrition

Nutrition is the science of foods, their components called nutrients, and the relationship between food, health and disease.

The first half of this book discussed the relationship of the hormones involved in appetite and the interferences from our environments that alter our ability to metabolize what we eat and how we eat. The science of appetite is so new that scientists are only now disseminating information and finding natural, healthy solutions like bauhinia to the Globesity epidemic. Our next discussion regarding eating serves two purposes:

• To help you make better food choices based upon the science you now know.

• To eat for health and longevity, as hard as it may be to keep your future in front of you instead of taste preferences.

Classes of Nutrients

There are six essential classes of nutrients, and a single class is determined by the function of the nutrient. Vitamins, minerals, and microminerals are considered micronutrients as they provider no energy to the body, thus we need very small amounts.

1. **Carbohydrates'** grouping includes sugars, starches and fibers. Natural sugars are found in fruits, honey, vegetables, and dairy foods (watch for glycemic index). Natural starch exists in vegetables and grains, the staple diet of our globe. Fiber refers to the plant material that passes through our digestive track without breaking down, cleaning the colon and preventing constipation. You may have experienced fiber when eating raw carrots, whole grains or nuts.

2. **Proteins,** as nutrients, replace amino acids that our body needs, replenish proteins as they break down and also build muscle and strength. Most of us eat more protein than we need, and the excess is used for energy. Eating excess protein does not equate into building muscle, and the kidneys are the main organs for processing protein wastes. Kidneys require much water to do their job. Like all nutrients, consume moderate protein in a balanced diet. Reconsider high-protein diets and your ability to manage protein. Remember to drink a lot of water to deal with a high protein diet to neutralize all that excess acid.

3. Fats & oils of certain types are needed by the body for growth and maintenance. Fats are also called lipids, a class of organic compounds, which do not dissolve in water. Good fats are "essential fatty acids" like omega-3. Cholesterol is a fat, but it is also made by our own body and is not considered an essential nutrient in our diet, but it is a critical component in every cell, hormone, and brain.

4. Minerals are basic elements that cannot be broken down. The body requires at least 45 known minerals. How many more of the 100 micro-minerals we need is unknown. The body uses minerals for conducting electricity, regulating chemical reactions, and providing structural components to the body.

5. Vitamins support all metabolic functions and are critical to metabolism, that is, creating energy. We need vitamins in small amounts to regulate chemical reactions.

6. Water is the most likely nutrient for sustaining human life. Water lubricates joints, transports nutrients, wastes, and regulates body temperature. Basically, water provides the medium for all the chemical activity in the body.

DOCTOR TAI'S IMPORTANT TIP

Keeping A Food Diary

To know how to develop a healthier lifestyle, first keep a food diary to determine your level of calories and nutrients as well as the balance of your intake from the food groupings.

One study from Kaiser Permanente's Center for Health Research found that keeping a food diary doubled the weight loss for the 1700 persons in the study, which was one of the first to include large numbers of African Americans. The average weight loss among the group was thirteen pounds, based upon a low fat diet rich in fruits and vegetables and with moderate exercise or levels of activity. [63]

[63] Public Press Release. "Kaiser Permanente study finds keeping a food diary doubles weight loss. (July 8, 2008) by Kaiser Permanente.

FOOD DIARY

(Fill in here ALL the foods you eat daily)

Date	Time	Food	Calorie Count	Portion	Reason to Eat

Chapter Twenty Five

EAT FOR ENERGY

Only One Reason To Eat!

Our eating is influenced by such diverse factors as habit, culture and social settings, so our choice to eat for energy and health may seem simple. We eat for one reason—energy!

Three of the nutrients' groups—carbohydrates, lipids and proteins—provide the energy for our metabolism.

These three groups are called **macronutrients** because bodies need large quantities, whereas vitamins and minerals are **micronutrients** because we need less. **So meal planning includes the energy producing foods.** Vitamins and minerals are supplements to your lifestyle's energy intake and expenditure.

The energy available from food is calories, and nutritionists suggest that a portion of your diet each day come from different food groups to provide your energy. For example, in the previous chapter, we discussed that the numbers of calories you ingest each day might be between 1200 and 1500 for a weight loss diet. Your fat intake would be 35% of the total caloric intake.

☞ *Fat Cells: Obese people and you have the same number of fat cells; the difference is the size of these fat cells. You don't become overweight because you make more fat cells...but the fat globules swell each fat cell and increase your body size.*

Carbohydrates

When doctors and scientists discuss **glucose** in our blood and its relationship to health, they speak not of table sugar, but the resulting molecule of eating, digesting and absorbing carbohydrates—sugars, fiber and starches. Whether we have fruits, whole grains, vegetables or milk products, the primary role of glucose is to circulate in our blood and provide energy to cells. Also, the body needs glucose to burn fat efficiently.

After eating, our bodies use glucose immediately to balance levels in the blood. Cells require small carbohydrate amounts to break down fat to release energy. Blood glucose that is too low makes someone feeling shaky and weak. High glucose levels leaves a person feeling sluggish and unfocused.

DOCTOR TAI'S IMPORTANT TIP

Weight Control Tips: *Take L-carnitine approximately* **3 grams a day** *to help muscles to be more efficient in the use of carbohydrates.*

Taking 2 to 3 gelcaps of Omega 3- 20 minutes before each meal satisfies the satiety factor.

Blood pressure and waist sizes are the best indicators of health problems.

Fructose blunts the satiety center because it tricks your mind so you stay hungry and continues to eat.

Your metabolism is dependent on your Thyroid and Liver.

Polycystic Ovary Syndrome (PCOS) is responsible for weight gain in about 20 percent of women.

A small bowl of Fiber fills you up and slows down the transit time of the gut.

The best strategy for waist control is to walk twenty to thirty minutes daily.

Your brain, the stomach, and small intestines regulate your weight control.

Glycemic Index

The glycemic rating of a food is a way for us to determine the speed with which glucose from foods enters the blood stream. Why is this important?

The more quickly glucose is absorbed causes a rapid increase in blood sugar, to which insulin and other hormones respond with a spike. The higher glycemic number associated with a specific food, the faster its glucose moves into the blood stream. A food, like protein with a lower number, is digested slowly and goes into the blood stream progressively.

Besides looking at foods with low numbers, also consider these facts when choosing food for weight loss factors:

• Processed animal products with added carbs like bacon and lunchmeats. Avoid these.

• Some low glycemic foods also contain a lot of unhealthy fat, which we do not want. These could be fatty meats, portions of pork and lamb, as well as poultry like duck. Dairy products fit into this category also. Choose a lean and low fat…low glycemic foods.

• While raw non-sweet fruits are low on the scale (blueberries, strawberries, raspberry), cooking fruit breaks down the sugar, for a higher level.

• Basically avoid any high fat, high carbohydrates foods.

• *Stay away from any foods not in existence 100 years ago!*

GLYCEMIC INDEX CHART

FOOD CATEGORIES	SUB-FOODS – RATING

SUGARS

Fructose - 20
Glucose - 100
Honey 32-87, average 55
Lactose 46
Sucrose (granulated table sugar) most 62

DAIRY PRODUCTS

Milk, regular (full fat) 11-40, average 27
Milk, skim - 32
Yogurt without added sugar - 14-23

CARBOHYDRTAES - CEREALS

Cold Cereal
All-Bran - 30-51, average 42
Bran Buds - 58
Bran Buds with Psyllium - 47
Cornflakes 72-92, average 81
   (USA cornflakes were the 92)
Corn Chex 83
Crispix 87
Fruit Loops - 69
Golden Grahams - 71
Grape Nuts - 71
Life - 66
Puffed Wheat - 67-80
Rice Krispie type cereals - 81-95
Rice Chex - 89
Shredded Wheat - 67-83 average 75
Special K - 54-84
Total - 76

Hot Cereal
Cream of Wheat - 66
Instant Cream of Wheat - 74
Oatmeal from rolled oats (not instant) - 58
Quick cooking oats - 66

Grains - Boiled Whole unless stated otherwise
Barley - 25
Barley, cracked - 50
Barley, rolled - 66
Buckwheat - 49-63
Cornmeal boiled in water - 69

Couscous (processed wheat) - 61-69
Millet - 71
Rice, long-grained white - 56
Rice, short and medium
  grained white – 88
Rice, brown - 55
Wheat, whole kernels - 30-48
Wheat, bulgar (cracked wheat) – 48

BREADS, MUFFINS CRACKERS

White bread 64-87 - averages 70 and 73
Whole wheat bread made with
  whole wheat flour - 52-87 average 71
Wheat bread made with 50% cracked
  wheat kernels 58
Wheat bread made with 75% cracked
  wheat kernels 48

**Muffins, Cakes, Pancakes,
Waffles, Bagels**
Vary widely (38-102), but most
  between 55 and 80

Crackers
Rice Cakes - 61-91, average 78
High fiber rye crispbread - 64
Stoned Wheat Thins – 6

FRUIT & FRUIT JUICES

Apples - 28-44, average 38
Raw Apricots - 57
Apricots, canned in light syrup - 64
Dried Apricots - 31
Apricot fruit spread (reduced sugar) - 55
Banana, overripe - 52
Cantaloupe – 65
Cherries - 22
Dates – 103
Grapefruit - 25
Grapes - 46-49
Kiwi - 54
Mangoes - 55
Oranges - 44
Papayas - 58
Peaches - 43
Pears - 38

Pineapple - 64
Plums – 39
Prune - 33
Raisins - 64
Strawberries - 40
Watermelon - 72

Fruit Juice
Carrot Juice - 43
Cranberry Juice Cocktail - 52-68
Grapefruit Juice 48
Orange Juice 46-53
Pineapple Juice - 46
Tomato Juice – 38

VEGETABLES & LEGUMES

Starchy Vegetables
Beets 64
Carrots 16-92 average 47
Corn 37-62, average 53
Parsnips 97
Peas, green, fresh or frozen – 48
Potato - in high 80's
Potato, instant - 80
Rutabaga 72
Sweet potato\yam - 61

Legumes - refers to cooked fresh legumes. Canned legumes have a higher rating
Black-eyed peas 33-50
Butter beans 28-36, average 31
Chick peas (garbanzo beans) 31-36
Chick peas, canned 42
Kidney beans 13-46, average 34
Kidney beans, canned 52
Lentils 18-37
Lentils, canned 52
Navy beans (white beans, haricot) 30-39
Navy beans, pressure cooked 29-59
Peas, dried, split 32
Pinto beans 39
Pinto beans, canned 45
Soy beans 15-20
Soy beans, canned – 14

Healthy, Nutritious Eating

• Recommended guidelines suggest that **carbohydrates comprise 30%** of your diet.

• Choose as often as possible natural and organic carbohydrates, whether raw or cooked: **non sweet fruits, vegetables and whole grains.**

• Two cups of each would provide about 1800 to 2000 calories when menu planning. Remember, salads count, one medium apple is approximately one cup of fruit. A small portion of legumes counts.

• Choose these foods for color variety also as dark green, orange-yellow, purple, red and so forth.

• The best cooking methods to maintain nutrients and enzymes for fruits and vegetables are **steaming, sauteing or blanching.**

• At least two-thirds of your grains should be whole grains like oats, brown rice, white rice, barley, millet or quinoa. Breads, muffins and bagels are not considered whole grains.

• Choose dairy products on the basis of your ability to digest them, and limit your intake as they produce mucous. **One-third of all Americans are allergic to pasteurized milk products.**

DOCTOR TAI'S IMPORTANT TIP

Exercise - *When you lose weight without exercise, you lose both muscle and fat, but when you gain weight without exercise, you gain only fat. It's easier to gain fat weight than it is to gain muscle weight, which is one of the reasons why "yo-yo" dieting fails. When you continually gain and lose and gain and lose, you end up gaining proportionally even fatter, because of the muscle loss.*

Chapter Twenty Six

BALANCING FOODS

How Much Fat?

Losing weight means that we will lose water, fats, and possibly lean mass like muscles. Lipids, the basic building blocks of fat, are in every cell, and fat contains little water. Fats from animal and vegetable sources provide a concentrated source of energy; provide the building blocks for cell membranes and a variety of hormones. Fats, as part of a meal, slow absorption so that we can go longer without feeling hungry.

 *Our bodies need **friendly fat like omega-3** to help keep cells hydrated. Without them, saturated fats fill the space within the cells, creating imbalance. (Not during Stage II diet)*

Deficiencies of essential fatty acids have been linked to a wide range of common disorders including:
- Heart and respiratory difficulties
- Hypertension
- Elevated LDL cholesterol
- Elevated triglycerides
- Insulin resistance (leading to type II diabetes)
- Memory Loss

Get half of the fats from monosaturated fats which are plentiful in olive oil, canola oil, almonds, avocado, walnuts… eat in moderation as fat is concentrated. Very small amounts of virgin coconut oil can actually assist with weight loss because it contains medium chain fatty acids or medium chain triglycerides (MCTs for short). The predominant MCT in virgin coconut oil is lauric acid.

We must consume a diet that provides animal foods rich in protective fats and vitamin B6 and B12. We must bolster thyroid function via the intake of good fats as well as through the use of natural sea salt that supplies an array of ocean micro-minerals as well as a usable source of organic iodine.

> ## Defending Fat
> The good side of fat is that it provides excellent insulation. Your fat is stored throughout your body as an energy reservoir. Brown fat (BAT) and is found inside protective areas of the body. It increases when you work outdoors during the winter to insulate vital organs. Adults have little brown adipose tissue (BAT). One-third of fat in babies is brown fat, which keep them warm and toasty. Brown fat is **different because it has blood vessels and nerves,** and it also has leptin receptors. Brown fat is more thermogenic, meaning it can break down excess calories into heat, with higher level of leptin.

Omega-3 fatty acid helps our bodies by decreasing inflammation like arthritis. More than a dozen studies have demonstrated that omega-3 fish oils can reduce arthritic symptoms and other inflammatory conditions. Mercury-free wild fish (if there are any left) are the best food for omega-3s. Other choices are oysters, omega-3 fortified eggs, flaxseeds, walnuts, plankton and seaweed.

Proteins

Proteins are nutritional workhorses and are the building blocks for muscle, bones, cartilage, skin, some hormones and all of our enzymes. Protein also helps regulate pH balance and formulate hormones and antibodies. In addition, enzymes, the managers and catalysts of all our biochemical processes, are specialized proteins. Our intestines break down the proteins we ingest into amino acids.

Of the **22 necessary amino acids**, our bodies manufacture 13, and foods supply the rest. Eight are considered essential nutrients. When these 8 essential amino acids are present, the body is capable of building the remaining nonessential amino acids on its own. If even one essential amino acid is low or missing, however, the body will be unable to synthesize the other proteins it needs.

Fibers

There are two types of fiber. Soluble fiber, which dissolves in water, is in legumes, barley, oats, variety of beans and most fruits. It shows a binding effect in the colon, moving bile and acids out of the body.

The second is insoluble fiber, mostly in whole grains and some stringy vegetables, forms a gel like substance. It increases stool bulk and helps pass wastes.

People who consume fiber-rich diets feel less hungry and ingest fewer calories during the day. High fiber foods cause one to eat slowly as they require chewing, thereby aiding digestion.

DOCTOR TAI'S IMPORTANT TIP

Recommended Daily Intake

38 grams of Fiber per day for men, and 25 grams per day for women up to age 50 help your digestion. Over age fifty persons should aim for an average of 30 grams daily. Increase fiber intake gradually to accommodate the intestinal fluctuations. Do not believe that more is better. A high fiber intake interferes with vitamin and mineral absorption. You absolutely need large amounts water to clear fiber out of the body.

Vitamins & Minerals

Only 5% of the human body is mineral matter, yet minerals are vital to mental and physical functions. Calcium, magnesium, sodium, potassium and iron are especially important for sending messages via the nervous system, digestion and metabolism and using other nutrients.

Minerals carry electrical current through the body; they are electrical conductors, so to speak. Every function of our body is electrical.

These micronutrients, vitamins, power the body's biochemical processes and activate the enzymes to ignite metabolism (Craving Factor is an excellent source). Vitamins and minerals also fight disease and repair tissue. The body does not assimilate vitamins without minerals…

- Vitamin C needs calcium
- Vitamin A needs zinc
- B vitamins need magnesium
- Vitamin E needs selenium

Vitamins, like fiber, are water-soluble and fat-soluble.

Water Soluble Vitamins Not stored in body and must be replaced frequently	Fat Soluble Vitamins Are stored in body and required less frequently	
Vitamin C	Vitamin A	Vitamin E
All B vitamins	Vitamin D	Vitamin K

Supportive Research

> *A study released in the spring, 2008 by the Agricultural Research Service suggests that plant foods help preserve muscle mass in older men and women.*

Researchers reviewed the kinks between measures of lean body mass and diets high in potassium-rich, alkaline-producing fruits and vegetables. "Based on regression models, volunteers whose diets were rich in potassium could expect to have 3.6 more pounds of lean tissue mass than volunteers with half the higher potassium intake. That almost offsets the 4.4 pounds of lean tissue that is typically lost in a decade in healthy men and women aged 65 and above."[64]

Cortisol-Lowering Vitamin & Mineral Supplements

Green tea extract, bitter orange peel, ginseng, passionflower, magnolia bark, citrus aurantium, beta-sitoserol, chromium, jujube fruit, and vanadyl sulfate.

---

[64] US Department of Agriculture (2008, May 31). Plant Foods For Preserving Muscle Mass. ScienceDaily. Retrieved December 28, 2008,

Chapter Twenty Seven

Dr. Tai's Asian Diet

If you fail to plan, then you plan to fail.

A Diet of Common Sense

I am happy to see the new diet books available in the last several years. *Feed Your Tiger: The Asian Diet Secret for Permanent Weight Loss and Vibrant Health*[65] by Hadady takes four animal symbols, dragon, bear, crane and tiger, which are plentiful in Asian art, to represent **the energy type** for specific eating protocols and slimming exercises.

Another book, *The Asian Diet: Get Slim and Stay Slim the Asian Way* by Tran, who grew up in Vietnam, introduces a blend of Asian and French techniques. The staples the author describes include rice, fish and seafood, sauces, primarily of fish and blending oyster sauce and soy, and many vegetables, fruits and teas…green, jasmine, chrysanthemum, and lotus.

What you may not see in Asian diets are milk or dairy products because many Asians do not have adequate lactase enzymes.

Enzymes Are Mandatory

 Enzymes *are large protein molecules, as well as a co-enzyme, which is usually a vitamin or mineral. These construction workers of the body's metabolic activity convert food into energy.*

All cultures have specific foods high in enzymes that aid in digestion. For example, when eating in a Japanese restaurant, your Miso soup is a digestive aid. Miso is a fermented food and breaks down other foods we eat for easier digestion.

---

[65] Hadady, L. *Feed Your Tiger: The Asian Diet Secret for Permanent Weight Loss and Vibrant Health.* Emmaus, PA: Rodale Books, (December 12, 2006)

Other cultures have enzyme-rich foods such as fermented dairy products like yogurt and kefir, fermented cabbage as sauerkraut and fermented soy like tempeh. In tropical countries, papaya and mango have high concentrations of enzymes, and have been used traditionally for the topical treatment of burns and wounds.

DOCTOR TAI'S IMPORTANT TIP

Fermented Appetizers: *The fermentation process helps release vitamins and minerals already present in the nutrient rich raw vegetables. Here are some of my favorites: pressed cabbage and red pepper salad, pickles, small helping of sauerkraut, light helping of greens with oil and vinegar, wasabi paste, fermented ginger, kim chee, or a small bowl of white Miso soup.*

Simple & Elegant Soup

In the Asian diet plan, start your meals with 12 to 14 ounces, or one bowl, of clear soup/broth. The broth is made of chicken, beef, pork or seafood bouillon, and then garnished with a medley of chopped seasonal vegetables. These soups are not based on any dairy ingredients like milk or cream, nor are they creamy, thick soups. The point of having soup first is to offer appetite relief, curbing hunger.

Research shows that soup is effective in a diet for weight loss because it reduces calorie consumption. "The link between eating soup and weight control is documented in a first-ever compendium of peer-reviewed science demonstrating that low energy-dense foods, like soup, can be an effective – and nourishing – part of any weight-management plan." [66]

---

[66] "Research Shows Eating Soup Can Be A Simple Strategy for Weight Management." Press release (January, 5, 2009) of study, *Soup as a Weight Management Strategy: A Comprehensive Research Review*," at www.CampbellSoup.com

Main Course

For the main course, have a variety of lightly cooked, steamed, or sautéed vegetables. The average person eats no more than 3 fingers of very thinly sliced meat or seafood (which makes it appear like a lot) accompanied by a large portion of 2-3 cups of vegetables.

Of course, we finish with one more bowl of vegetables or clear soup.

Flavorful Choices

Variety and food rotation keep your taste buds interested! Today, you might modify this meal by choosing soup with a large salad mixed with a variety of vegetables of different colors, texture, and flavors. Tomorrow you might jazz up your salad with eggs, thinly sliced meats, or seafood. Sprinkle with nuts, tomatoes, beans and onions if you like.

More flavorful selections include grated fresh ginger, chopped green onions, grated carrots, sliced zucchini or summer squash, bok choy chopped in chunks or sliced thin like cabbage.

- Snow peas complement thin sirloin beef strips well.
- Garlic cloves and thinly sliced sweet onions add aroma and aid digestion.
- Sliced or grated ginger, in the smallest pinch, adds flavorful digestive support, especially with spinach and mushrooms

Light Dressings

Be mindful of salad dressings! Keep them simple and light. The best dressings are made with cold-pressed extra virgin olive oil, lemon juice with a little zest, or Mirin or rice wine vinegar, which plays an important role in enhancing the digestive enzyme in your stomach. This is a very important part of the diet; as we get older, our stomachs do not make as much acid as is needed for digestion.

> **Variations of Sesame Oil Dressings**
> *Light sesame oil is delicious on steamed or blanched vegetables like green beans. Toasted sesame oil offers a smoky flavor. Mix 1 tablespoon of shoyu to the sesame oil and sprinkle lightly on a spinach leaves and purple onion salad. Add a third ingredient, two teaspoons of rice vinegar for a tangy taste.*

Desserts

Lastly, a typical dessert, in small portion, is a medley of different fresh fruits cut in cubes. Do not follow the typical American habit of buying a single fruit like watermelon and eating it completely in a sitting. Small amounts of different fruits make a fresh fruit salad with more variety, more color, and more taste--with heavy emphasis on blueberries, raspberries, and strawberries. Your meal will be delightfully complete, clean, and light.

Eating this way, you can easily lose 2 pounds a month. That's 24 pounds a year!

My Personal Secret - Dr. Tai's Story

I follow mostly all the supplements, **The Thin Factors, Craving Factor, Slimming Lyposome , Max Metabolism, Super B 12** *and the 3 gelcaps Omega3 before every meal.*

I recommend in this book, in addition to dietary foods, one 4-hour period of no food. Start this routine of closing the kitchen at 8 PM and do not open it again until morning.

The Asian Diet is my secret for weight loss. I lost 50 pounds in two to three years. Today, I weigh 140 pounds, have less than 10% body fat and have a 29-inch waist on a 5-foot, 11-inch frame. My body weight is set and kept the same weight for years.

That's a reasonable weight I can live with and maintain. That means in a weak moment, if I fall off the wagon for two days, I get right back and tighten the dietary reins for a week. Voila! I am back on track. It has become a lifestyle...NO EFFORT!!!

I know it can be for you too...GOOD LUCK and GOOD HEALTH!!! Cheers...

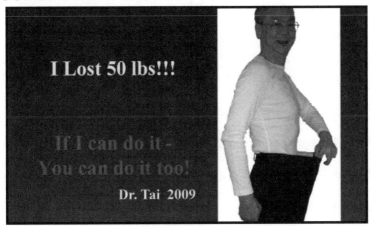

STAGE I

1200 calorie Diet – Low Carb, No Sugar, Low Fat - 30 Days

* You must drink 5 bottles of 16oz. of fluid daily
to wash away your fat.
(2 in the morning, 2 in the afternoon, and one at night.)
* Keep a diary of your food intake each day – Don't cheat
on your calorie counts!
* Plan your meal ahead, Eat on a set schedule &
Eat before you get hungry

Supplements

1. **The Thin Factors**- Two capsules 15-30 minutes before you
   eat 3x daily, even if you are skipping a meal.

2. **Max Metabolism** - . Two capsules before each meal. 3x
   daily, even if you are skipping a meal.

3. **Craving Factor** - Dissolve 1 teaspoon in 8-16 ounces of
   breakfast, throughout the day and again in the evening
   before dinner. (drink 5 bottles a day)

4. **The Slimming Fat Burn Cream- 7-Keto** - Scientifically
   Backed Active Ingredient. Rub 3-4 pumps on areas needed
   help to lose inches, AM & PM.

5. **Weight & Inches** - One capsule a half an hour before eating.

6. **Max Performance** – One tablet 3x daily with food.

7. **Super B12** – Three sprays AM & Noon.

8. **Max Sea** – 15 drops with water twice daily.

STAGE II

500 calorie Diet – Only for 40 Days! – No Sugar, No Fat, Low Carb.

*** You must drink 5 bottles of 16oz. of fluid daily
to wash away your fat.
(2 in the morning, 2 in the afternoon, and one at night.)
* Keep a diary of your food intake each day – Don't cheat
on your calorie counts!
* Plan your meal ahead, Eat on a set schedule & Eat
before you get hungry**

1. Continue with ALL of above Stage I supplements
2. Add: **Hunger Factor**, A Natural Hormone supplement -
   one dose AM & before dinner for 40 days that helps to reshape you to a younger body!

**Health Secrets USA
24141 Ann Arbor Trail, Dearborn Heights, MI 48127
PH: 313-561-6800 Fax: 313-561-6830**
www.healthsecretsusa.com   office@healthsecrets.com

INDEX

241